Food for Health and Cure

Food for Health and Cure

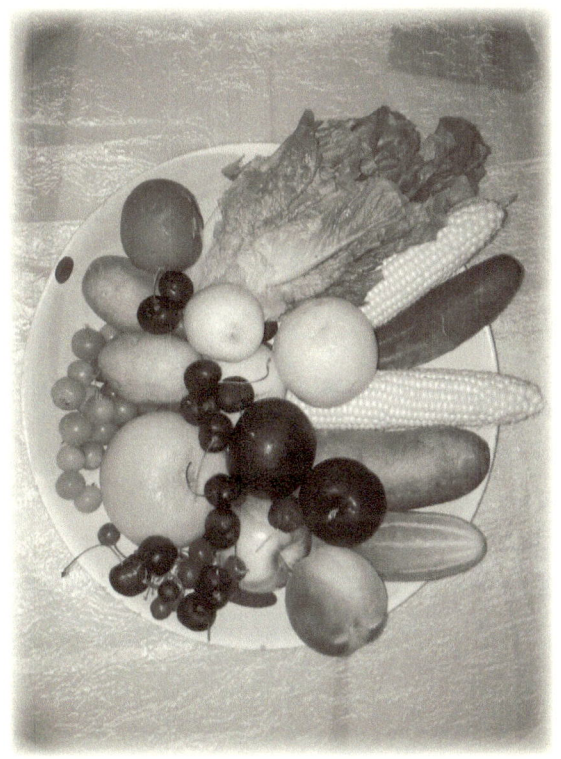

Marie F. Dubreuil

To order additional copies of this book, contact:
Xlibris
1-888-795-4274
www.Xlibris.com
Orders@Xlibris.com
670044

ACKNOWLEDGMENTS

Thanks to my grandson Charles Erick, a computer wizard who assisted me in all computer work such as organizing written material, e-mailing the book to the publisher, communicating with the publisher, traveling from North Carolina to New York to get this book out to the public and ready for the holidays.

Thanks to David, my computer technician at the beginning of the book, and thanks to Tom, my computer technician close to the end of the book, for helping with computer problems.

Thanks to my daughter Karen for advising me to stop writing book number 2 and to continue with the rest of my information in another book. Therefore, this book will come out sooner and be more portable.

INTRODUCTION

Knowledge is power.

This book gives everyone who read it the power to control their health!

How Does It Do That?

By telling everyone what food to eat for almost any illness or condition that people want to alleviate, eradicate, prevent, and cure. It also tells people about any food drawbacks, bad foods to stay away from and to cut down, depending on the person's needs. It is not possible to cover all foods good or bad and all diseases and conditions in one book. But it can only tell people the benefits and drawbacks for a large number of foods and illnesses.

Just like in the previous book name T.H.A.T.S. (The Health Assistance to Some), *people who read it can obtain the power to protect their foods against organisms and diseases. These organisms are the following: bacteria, virus, parasites, fungus, and mold. Meanwhile, this book,* Food for Health and Cure, *tells people about the foods that are good and bad for a large number of illnesses, diseases, or conditions that people can have, prevent, and cure.*

Food for Health and Cure *doesn't mean that people are going to stop every medical treatment or intervention and just rely on food alone for everything they have. People should continue to have their annual checkup, physical, follow-up, take their prescribed drugs and treatments from their doctors. As a matter of fact, in the medical profession, there is a diet for almost every disease and condition*

7

that people already have. Meaning that if people have this particular disease or condition, there are foods along with medical care that can help them to be cured, treated, or relieved faster than if they weren't eating this type of foods.

For example, if after their annual physical or checkup they are free from diseases but want to maintain their good health, there are foods that they can eat and food that they can't eat to do just that in this book. If on the contrary some people find out that they are sick, there is the probability that their illness can be hereditary, genetic, a precondition or they're just out of shape and aging prematurely. They will then know already what to eat or not for this particular situation or condition if it's in this book. People can more likely find almost all the common conditions in this book. I am pretty sure that if it's a rare condition that is not in this book the physician finding it or taking care of the patients would have a special diet for these patients.

Good food and good nutrition play a key role in people's life. Although there are a lot of sick people in this world, there are also some very healthy people who live a long life without touching drugs. Just knowing what food to eat and what food to stay away, to cut down, along with activity and other good advice in this book can make anyone a part of these drug-free, healthy, and happy people. The knowledge of good foods in this book can help everyone in any condition to do better, stay healthier, treated faster, stay younger, live longer, and be happier. What's great with good foods is that they pop up in a great many diets and conditions.

When I started this study, investigation, research, and data collection in 2006, I was amazed to find out that sometimes the same foods are good for so many illnesses and conditions. To me, some foods are like the mitochondria, the powerhouse, the source of energy in the cell, because these foods are involved in so many important processes, that is, protein synthesis and lipid metabolism and others. And also as a higher plan or a miracle, these same foods have less drawbacks. According to my investigation and to scientists, if some people are allergic to some good foods, they can find many other good foods to replace them.

The Benefits of Good Foods

Sometimes people don't have the knowledge of good foods to eat. No matter who they are, they can harm themselves. Good foods don't mean tasty in the *palate only; they also mean healthy in the arteries, heart, brain, pancreas, liver, stomach, intestines, lungs, and every organ inside and outside of the body. For the outside of the body, these foods that people eat good or bad can show in their look, appearance, shape, skin, hair, eyes, nails, height, width, walk, movement, speech, vision, behavior, mode, sensation, perception, alertness, vitality, energy, and intelligence. It's like the slogan for the commercial sauce: "Prego it's in there."*

In the United States, recently there is a former politician whom I know was probably eating for taste at a Southern restaurant where meals are the tastiest. I know this fact by experience from working for the State in Harlem.

My boss used to treat me with a take-out breakfast of grits, fried eggs, bacon, home fries, and biscuits. Other times, it was with lunch of brown rice and black-eyed peas, fried chicken, collard greens, and peach cobbler for dessert from the same restaurant. The foods were really delicious in the mouth, but not that great health wise. And that was due to the large amount of saturated fat, calories, and the preparation or cooking style. I know these facts from medical sciences, research, experiment, and experience.

Some of these foods served in that restaurant for breakfast were grits, eggs, bacon, and biscuits.

Grits, although a very starchy and high-calorie food, still could have been a healthy food and part of an important meal to start the day. But with all the animal products cooked with it—for example, fats from pork lard and butter—change it from healthy to bad food.

Eggs, any style, should be good for health if they were not cooked with butter, animal saturated fat, pork lard, hydrogenated, partially hydrogenated or trans fat. But the eggs served in that place were. On the contrary, the eggs could have been very healthy if they were cooked without oil, any other way but fried, or at least with natural vegetable oil.

Biscuits, made with whole wheat, whole grain of barley, sunflower seeds, pumpkin and flax seed, enriched flour, vegetable oil that's not hydrogenated or partially hydrogenated, no MSG, no saturated fat could have been a part of a healthy meal; but they were not.

Lunch was made of Southern fried chicken, collard greens, black-eyed peas, rice, peach cobbler.

Fried Chicken

If the chicken was all natural; organic; 97 percent fat free; free from a cage; free range; running around; without growth hormones, steroid antibiotics, and anti-anxiety for stress-induced tranquilizer and fatty animal products as feeding made for them artificially, it could have been an excellent meal rich in protein, enzymes, and vitamins and minerals. To me, chicken should be cooked any style except fry (rarely) to be good for health. On the contrary, this fried chicken was cooked fried with pork fat; lard; butter; hydrogenated, partially hydrogenated oil, or trans fat; high salt and sodium content; MSG with the potential of raising blood pressure; triglycerides; phospholipids; cholesterol (LDL), the fatty one, which burst your fat cells and send the entire body to "kingdom come" in a matter of months. Talking about LDL cholesterol, some scientists used to say that the LDL cholesterol was bad and causes heart attacks. But other new scientists recently discovered that the LDL cholesterol is not bad at all. It is just fatty, and other reasons caused heart attacks, which is just what I always believed.

Home Fried and French Fried Potato

Potato cooked in animal fat and its being a starch carbohydrate can put a toll on people's pancreas and liver. When fried in pork lard, beef fat, or trans fat, it becomes unhealthy. While if potato was cooked baked with vegetable oil with some skins or boiled, it could have been a healthy meal. The potato served in this restaurant was fried in animal fats. Potato is a root vegetable rich in potassium and other beneficial minerals and vitamins.

Peach Cobbler

This could have been a delicious dessert; because of all the vitamins and minerals, non-animal product, whole grain enriched flour, and its being partly fruit should make it a healthy food. But the butter as animal product, the lard, the saturated and trans fat oil, the white bleach and refined flour and all the chemicals and spices added to it for taste can easily turn this food to toxin and be unhealthy.

Collard Greens

Collard greens is a green leafy vegetable, which is full of fibers, vitamins, and minerals. The fibers make collard greens healthy for the arteries, lower cholesterol (LDL), the fatty one, and increase good cholesterol (HDL). It regulates bowel movement and is good for the digestive system and weight problems. Collard greens is cheap, keeps you full, and is low in calories. Collard greens contains the following vitamins: A, E, D, K, C, and some B. All of these vitamins are good for your blood cells, but the vitamin K that have been omitted and neglected by some people is the best.

In the medical field, people know that vitamin K is good for clotting, coagulation, and stopping or preventing bleeding. In most nursing schools overseas and in United States, the first IM (intramuscular) injection assigned to their students in maternity is a vitamin K solution given to the newborn baby in the largest muscle, which is the thigh for the United States and the buttocks for some other countries. This injection is to prevent bleeding after cutting the umbilical cord. Next is the tetanus shot to prevent the tetanus toxin or lockjaw, a deadly condition for newborn.

The Minerals

Adding to all the benefits of the vitamins, collard greens contains some minerals. Calcium, which is good for bones, nails, hair, skin and eyes, also alleviate your joint and bone pain. Iron can enrich the blood and prevent anemia.

Collard greens is a cabbage family that contains sulforaphane, which is good for many conditions. When cooked without pork fat, lard, animal oil or fat, saturated fat, trans fat, salt, brown sugar, and not boiled for too long, it retains the sulforaphane and all the vitamins and minerals. It can make a delicious and healthy dish. Collard greens should be steamed at medium heat and completely covered for fifteen minutes at the most. All one needs to add in collard greens are one tablespoon of olive oil or any natural vegetable oil, fresh garlic, and onion or powder or any seasoning of your choice that doesn't have the chemicals or additives that are provided in another chapter of this book.

Black-Eyed Peas

Black-eyed peas is a great source of fiber because it's a legume and beans family. The fibers in beans are components of food that are resistant to chemical digestion. These fibers include portions of food that are made of cellulose, hemicellulose, lignin, and pectin. These substances add bulk to the diet by absorbing a large amount of water. Fiber can produce a large bulky bowel movement. Foods rich in fiber include whole grain food, bran flakes, leafy vegetables, root vegetables and their skins, prunes, which also contain the laxative substance diphenyl isatin and SYN roughage. Therefore, collard greens and black-eyed peas with their fibers can help prevent diverticula of the intestinal tract, may help lower the bad cholesterol, and possibly prevent cancer of the intestinal tract. For some diabetic people on low insulin doses, fibers are able to lower (even more) their insulin requirements. It's possible for people with type 2 diabetes to only use a diet rich in fibers, such as vegetables, black beans, black-eyed peas, whole grains, brown and black rice, lean meat, fish, poultry, fat-free dairy or lean protein, no concentrated sweet except the sweet from fruits and cinnamon powder on their dessert and their tea, along with some exercises or activities and weight loss to make type 2 diabetes something in the past for some people.

Brown, Black, Red, Purple, and Wild Rice

They are all part of whole grains. And when cooked in combination of dry beans of any kind or in soup, it can make a healthy meal with complete protein. All that is needed to cook the rice are water, olive oil or vegetable oil, onion, or garlic, fresh or powder. Do not add salt, butter, lard, smoked meat or poultry, bacon, nor processed meat to the rice. The latter can turn the rice to an artery-clogging food instead of food for cure.

Conclusion with the Former Politician Eating Food for Taste and My Experience with Some Southern Foods

Although I liked to please my boss for the treats, I only tasted the food that was delicious and discarded the rest in the garbage where it belonged. I knew it was bad for my health. This food was almost like home made. It was like almost all Southern cooking with all the animal fats, the smoked meats, the beef fat, the pork lard, the butter, the accent, the salted meat, the fried vegetables and meats and poultries, which some Southern people are used to. Like it or not, it's bad for their health.

Going back to this politician, I am glad that he was lucky enough to pull through after an open-heart surgery and triple bypass and good eating habits of healthy foods, exercise, relaxation, and meditation. To be honest with you, I think eating in that restaurant that served all these fatty foods had a great deal to do with this man's conditions.

The Additives in the Foods

In this book, besides people with certain conditions and the foods that are good for them, you can also find the additives that are good or bad for their conditions also. For this reason, this book provides people with all the known additives in food and their signs or keys next to the additive's symbols. These are explained in detail in different parts of the book. That's why people must read labels on food packages. People need to know the reason for the additives, what they do for the food, good or bad.

This information is vital for people's well-being. Unless people start cooking their foods from scratch from some supermarket and farm and own a garden, they need to know what in their food packages are in order to be healthy. If people don't know and continue to eat bad foods full of chemicals or additives and organisms, they won't get better or be cured even with drugs, medical procedures, diets, and exercises.

For example, my husband and I noticed the same people walking in the same mall twice a day at the same time, for the same number of hours almost every day, and remaining the same in appearance. They have long arms and legs, big fat and compact torsos, short thick necks, large fat faces, big heads, big round protruded fat stomachs. They look like they never lost one pound from the start to the present time. While my husband and I were walking, we carried a conversation with some of them and found out that they don't cook for themselves and only eat already prepared foods from department stores and supermarkets, probably with all the wrong chemicals and additives in these foods. As a result, these people become part of the statistic of "change in appearance," which is wide, compact, and obese, just like my discovery in the other book T.H.A.T.S.

It is a fact that not too many people can or want to cook from scratch for themselves and their loved ones. So they have to be smart and knowledgeable enough to read labels, learn to recognize the additives and chemicals that foods contain. They have to know which one is to be decreased, stopped using, used with caution, permitted by the health department and which one with allergens. Remember, people can't just rely on the government alone to check and recheck and stop people from inventing and selling these additives or chemicals good or bad for people to eat. The government and the health department are so overwhelmed with that responsibility that we have to start helping ourselves with our foods. Some of these additives are beneficial to people. But most of them are not. The government can't test all of them to know for sure which one is bad or not too bad and very bad. It takes too much time, employees, and money to do the needed procedure. Just remember for a while: most of our foods come from a foreign country. The inventors of these additives and chemicals are making them so rapidly that it becomes impossible for the government's personnel to catch them in time or before they are in the foods and the markets for people to buy and eat them. People must realize that the people who invented these additives are making a lot of money from them and won't stop making them regardless of what they can do to people. Most of the time these people who manufactured, invented, or found these products, additives, or chemicals don't eat or use them in their foods. These people usually are rich and have their cooks and nutritionists in their mansions to prepare their food organically, naturally, and safely.

The question is, what can we do to avoid eating these bad additives and chemicals in our foods? We know they can make us sick!

The answer is in this book where people can learn to read labels with meaning. People must know what they are looking for when reading the labels. This book tells you in great details and explanations about all known additives and chemicals in the market, the known all-natural foods, the organic foods, and some conditions that some additives can give, correct, and aggravate. Also, people can learn about some foods that can prevent, ameliorate, cure, or worsen some conditions or illnesses that they have.

I discovered something wonderful, which is people don't have to eat a large amount of different foods for various conditions because for most of the conditions, people can eat the same foods. Or another way to say it is that people can have from five to ten different conditions and find a group of five to ten different foods that are good for their conditions. Meaning if people are eating one type of food for one condition, that same type of food can prevent or cure another condition that they already have or are going to have in the future. This book covered that finding in the chapter for diseases and conditions and foods for them good or bad.

A Journey Full of History and Mystery

Sitting down and eating a meal is like taking a journey that is full of history and mystery. It is up to you to make the journey pleasant, adventurous, risky, unknown, predictable or not, cultural, sociable, and beneficial or not. It all depends on your knowledge of foods, planning of the meals, and paying attention to foods in general. Do you ever ask yourself what part of this country or the world the foods that you eat come from? And once you ask this question to yourself or others, you are very close to discover the unknown, the mystery of the journey that you are taking every day that you eat a meal.

All you have to do is pay attention in order to discover many secrets, adventures, risks, beauty and ugliness, the good, the bad, and the worst and the best about your foods. While paying attention, you will learn enough to discover the whereabouts of the key to unlock the Pandora box or the treasure that can be your health or your sickness. Again with this knowledge that you acquired, it's up to you to empower yourself. Just read this book and pay attention to what you read and also to almost everything else in life.

Paying Attention to Food

Although some people are obsessed with foods and love foods so much that they can eat anything as long as it's named food, they don't usually pay enough attention to what they eat. Some people eat food to fill up their stomach, satisfy their hunger or craving, to please themselves and others, for comfort or taste. Other people eat because they have to in order to survive and don't really care about what they eat. Most people eat and don't even know about the foods they eat, can't even remember what they eat, when they eat, and why they choose that particular food. Most of the time, their answers when I questioned them were as follows: "Why do you choose that food?" "Hmm, let's see! Because it tastes good, it's delicious, the food make me feel good, great, and satisfied." "What did you eat today?" "I don't even remember what and when. I just grabbed something this morning on my way to work." One person told me, "Hold it; I remember I ate a whole roasted chicken from a department store." "Anything else with it?" "No, that's all."

When paying attention, just know that everything you do or don't can make a difference. When it comes to food, know that every little bite of food that you take can and will either help or hurt. But if the little bite is of a good food, continue taking it until you obtain the benefit that you expect from that food. Don't give up because of impatience. This good food for you which is in this book can make you healthier, live longer, or cure you. In the contrary, if you find out that a particular food can be bad for your health and it's proven in this book, drop it like a hot potato, like it or not. Please don't continue to eat something that can make you sick or prevent your cure just because you like the taste of that food.

Now you do have the choice. After you know what to eat for what you want to cure, prevent, get better or worse, the control is in your hands. The power becomes yours. Before the knowledge from this book, you had limited options. But now your options become limitless or infinite. Because we have so many good foods that we can eat for what we want; we can easily replace the bad foods with the good foods. And we need to eat good foods to be healthy. Don't forget that we are what we eat. This statement is a fact of life. And there is no doubt about it. Therefore, why don't we eat only the good foods for health, sick or not.

Paying attention in general is good for all of us. Paying attention is what keeps us safe, knowledgeable, alert, and smart. According to a survey I conducted in 2007, I had a revelation. I used to think that people who passed by a place almost every day for a major part of their lives knew what was in that place, for example, the streets, the businesses, subways, parks, entertainments, etc. After I got the result of my survey, I can see that I was very wrong. For this survey, I chose a semiresidential and commercial place in Brooklyn, New York, and a residential place in Massapequa, Long Island. And the result made no difference as far as paying attention.

The Result for Brooklyn

Out of the five hundred people, men and women from any age, young adults to senior citizens, only 5 percent were able to answer the entire questionnaire accurately. Some of the questions were the following: name four businesses, two subway stations, four medical buildings, and four corner streets to enclose the block that you pass by for five to ten years almost every day to go to work, shop, visit family and friends, and go to a medical facility.

Some of the answers were a dry cleaner, a beauty salon, a Chinese restaurant, and a hardware store.

The subways were Myrtle Avenue and Broadway.

The medical buildings were two hospitals and two nursing homes.

The streets were Broadway, Myrtle Avenue, Cedar Street, and Bushwick Avenue.

In the Long Island people survey, it was very difficult to find a large number of people in the street at any time. Although I went to the malls, train station, and neighborhood streets, I could only have a two hundred fifty sample, which failed badly. These people are less friendly, private, don't talk to strangers, don't even notice people that live five blocks away from them for twenty years. And they also don't know the streets around them after living in their home for fifteen to twenty years, especially the older people who barely leave their house after retirement. Probably, the younger population would know. But it was not directed to them.

Although their questions were different, they couldn't answer them accurately. Either because they don't know, didn't pay attention, or don't want to bother. I made believe that I was lost and want to find my way, which was three blocks away from the individuals I asked.

Where is the nearest mall? The answer was three blocks away from where I stopped my car to ask.

Where was the post office, which was at a corner two blocks away from where I asked?

Where were the streets named Ann Rose and Emily Ann, which were each two blocks away in opposite directions?

A few people sent me to Ann Rose in the direction for Emily Ann. These people were sincere enough to leave their house and stand in the street and point the opposite directions to me. They really didn't know after twenty years living in the same square block of these two streets.

The excuses for the people in the train station LIRR and the mall were legit because these people claimed that they don't live where the questions were asked. But for the others right there in their houses, it was a disaster.

My Recommendation

I recommend that people search, seek knowledge, know about food, and learn about what foods can do to you and for you, good and bad food. Sit down and think about foods before you even make your shopping list for foods to buy or to order at the restaurants. At home, make your daily menu before shopping and start cooking so you will know what you need to buy and what you already have.

In the restaurant from the menus already made for you, compose your own from different entrees of what you know are good for your health. Because you can almost never find everything compatible, healthy and good for you, in one single menu organized for you. Most of the time, you have to work it out to your healthy satisfaction. Remember, usually what is tasty in your mouth is not good for your health. What is easy to prepare is not healthy for you to eat. What is healthy for you to eat most of the time take longer to prepare. What you like to eat is not what provides you with energy, natural nutrients, vitamins, and minerals that your body needs. What is good in your stomach, fill you up real fast, and calm down your hunger is not what your body needs at all.

Most of the time, the sugary, fatty donuts; the creamy pastries; the cakes; the thick shakes are made with white bleached flour, refined white sugar, high fructose corn syrup, or artificial chemical sugar substitute or man-made in the laboratories, which are poisons. Next comes the type of fats: animal saturated fats, whole milk, heavy cream, fatty cheese, butter, lard, trans fats, or hydrogenated or partially hydrogenated fat in vegetable oils, which are definitely bad for any one's health. Furthermore, the smoked ham, pig's feet, fried pork or fried meats in general, salty and smoky meat, smoky and salty poultry, fish, the bacon, the pastrami and all the preservatives, the dye and the processed food, the white potatoes, white rice, and food made with bleached flour including breads and pastas can take a big toll on your pancreas and your liver. The above foods can cause a host of diseases such as cardiovascular problems, heart attacks, stroke, cancer, diabetes, high blood pressure, high cholesterol, LDL, obesity, depression, and Alzheimer's. They could also change your appearance or keep you out of shape and cause anger, aggression, rage, and temporary psychosis.

Therefore, when you don't know about food, don't eat too much of any food. A simple option during the summer can include several pieces of watermelon and a bottle of spring water to cover your electrolyte needs.

Remember that anything done excessively can harm you. Eating good foods moderately can prevent or help until you find a cure or may even cure you of many diseases or conditions if the foods are appropriate for what you have.

Some foods are full of adrenaline producers, enhancers, energy boosters that lift or boost, hyper upper, picker upper, downers, sexual performance increaser, mood elevator, subdue, anesthetic, lethargic, sleep inducer, or stay awake. Some of the foods' side effects are known to almost everyone. But that does not stop some people from eating them excessively at the wrong time. For example, foods that contain caffeine should not be eaten close to sleeping time. And some animal protein food with tryptophan, melatonin, endorphin, which are sleep inducers, should not be eaten when you need energy to stay awake. People still indulge in these foods at the wrong time and with the wrong reasons. Maybe they don't know.

You Are What You Eat

Some people voluntarily or involuntarily eat too much of foods that can produce aggression and mood swings or ingest animal hormones through eating the drug in the animals as food. Don't forget that we are what we eat. And now, with all the steroids and growth hormones given to the animals to make them grow fast, grow big, adding to the aggressive nature of some animals before the drug, this can really be devastating. For example, you have the bull, which is very aggressive by nature, some fish or seafood, some birds, wild boars, deer, which are usually aggressive animals. And guess what? Some people eat them all. And again, we are what we eat. By eating these vicious animals, we behave like them sometimes. Now you can see the new trend in the USA, which is killing animals and people. All killings are bad, but some killings are the worst. To me, the number one bad killing is killing a police officer. Police officers or law enforcers should be respected, admired, and appreciated for the risky, life-threatening, and dedicated job they do to protect us during the days, nights, 365 days, 24 hours and 7 days a week, against the bad people. Therefore, law enforcement is my number 1 profession.

When I am walking in the streets, if I cross an officer or a group of officers, it is an honor for me to smile and say, "Hi, how are you" and "Have a nice day or evening." Sometimes, if I am on the other side opposite to them, I make it my duty to cross over to the police officer's side to say hi. When I think about these people leaving their beds, cozy homes, and their loved ones at home to risk their lives in the hot and cold nights and days year-round just to protect us, I don't see it as their jobs or a way of making a living. I see it as a commendable profession because they could have chosen something else to do.

My number two are the firefighters who deserved the same attention and admiration as number one.

My number three are the medical professionals: doctors, nurses, nurse aides, psychologists, radiologists, technicians, pathologists, biologists, epidemiologists, social workers, etc., are doing a great job for other people.

My number four are good lawyers, which can be like good doctors; they are great too when they save the good guys falsely accused and get the real bad guys.

My number five are teachers. They are commendable too because without them, there wouldn't be the president, the politicians, and all the rest of us. All the people above are appreciated greatly by me and others too for doing their job even if it is not 100 percent of their ability sometimes. I am 95 percent sure that they have a choice of professions and they are not doing what they do just for the money but because they like to do it.

My number six are the politicians, starting with the president, the vice president, the senators, the governors, the mayors, etc. They have a big responsibility and can't even sleep at night from worrying. They are people who need to be respected too.

My number seven are the news reporters, communications people such as in TV, newspaper, and radio who provide us with what is going on throughout the country and the world. They are useful, commendable, and brave people that should be respected too by us.

The servicemen, who are my number eight and who put their lives in danger to fight for our freedom overseas, leaving their loved ones behind, to me are so brave and need to be respected and admired too.

My number nine are the entertainers who can make us laugh, sing along, dance, and take an imagining journey through the wonderland, an oasis full of happiness, and get us out of our misery of bill collectors, unemployment, poverty, illnesses and diseases, bad relationships, and a crime-laden world.

My number ten are the farmers who provide foods for us to eat and survive, be strong, energetic and healthy; they are respectable people too.

My number eleven are the architects and construction workers who build bridges for the transportation of goods and people and also houses to live in; they are admirable and commendable people too.

My number twelve are the scientists and inventors who work restlessly to find new cures, new technology, new gadgets and trinkets, means of communication, transportation, space programs, medications, and surgical procedures. They are exceptional people and need to be respected and admired also.

There are a lot of other people in other good professions who need to be admired, commended, and respected too. But I can only name a few for space and move on.

Long ago, people were not as bad as they are now. They were not so sick and so big either as they are in some parts of the world and the USA. Most people used to work on the farm; raise horses, cows, chicken; have dairies; and make products that were natural and healthy. People were not so much after money to cage animals and use growth hormones, fertilizers, and fatty feeds for animals. People could wait for the foods to grow naturally on time. They used to have small farms with more people to take care of the foods grown on the ground without fertilizer or chemicals. The animals for food used to be free to move around, eat grass, and take their time to grow naturally without growth hormones, steroids, antibiotics, and chemicals. There used to be small farms and not so many big corporations and a lot of machines, cages, and fatty artificial foods to make them sick and drugs to cure them.

Even professionals used to exchange services for foods with people who couldn't pay them with money. At present, not only would people not give their services before obtaining the money, sometimes they take the money first and not give the services. Other times, they give the services and not get paid or receive the money and have to go to court to get paid or to give the services. In this century, some people are so inclined toward making money that they forget their health, which can be the least of their priority. Recently in the United States, a millionaire is no longer a big deal. The billionaire is what is in style. In this country, some people give their clothes, nails, hairstyle, cars or vehicles, and homes more attention and priority than foods for health. Some people spend hours doing their nails, hair; applying fragrance, makeup; trying on clothing; shopping for shoes, handbags, cars, jewelry, etc.; and have an empty refrigerator at home, buying reduced and outdated foods, food in bulk and auction, or take five minutes to cook meat and poultry, seafood and fish, or rush to a fast-food restaurant to eat. Most of these fast-food restaurants serve fatty burgers and fried and carbonated sweet drinks that these people gobble down in no time. After that, they run nonstop to somewhere except home to a cooked meal prepared by a family member or themselves. People should sit down by the table and eat a good home-made, well-cooked, full-of-vitamins, delicious, nutritious, and protected meal with family members. And after that, they should relax with loved ones and enjoy their good health.

Talking about protected food, today, Thursday, September 24, 2009, I watched on the news of channel 7 ABC about food delivered from the wholesale markets to the restaurant after three hours under a temperature of ninety-six degrees Fahrenheit, in a truck that was not refrigerated. These foods were animal products, such as beef, chicken, sour cream, milk, eggs, butter, and cheese, which were under a cold temperature of forty-five degrees Fahrenheit or above, which was the danger zone according to the reporter. This reporter said that he was going to report these trucks' business drivers to the health department to do something about this dangerous process. This proved what I said in my other book T.H.A.T.S. about eating out in the restaurants instead of your own cooking at home with the food protection knowledge. Please cook your food without risk by following what you learn from my book. Otherwise, you can have food poisoning that can be dangerous and fatal sometimes.

People should also take time to entertain friends and family by watching sports, movies, educational shows on TV or just listen to music. You can do these things alone too. Almost nobody does these things anymore. They rather run to a restaurant, order on the phone some unknown foods, and hurry up to go to job number 1 or job number 2 if they still have even one to make money. All the above are something in the past for some people.

Be Careful about Some Dieters

For the past few years, because of the obesity epidemic, this country became full of weight-reducing diet makers. Some of them are legit, but others are not. Most of the time, some people without medical knowledge just join the bandwagon to make money. Even some of the best-seller dieters tell people to cook their turkey breast or turkey burgers sautéed in a sauce pan for five minutes. This best seller is one of the most reputable and well-known diets makers tell people about the most unhealthy meals composed with foods that can make them sick in a few hours. Yes, if the person survives the bad foods treatment, there is a possibility that this person can drop a few pounds and a few inches or two to three clothing sizes. But guess what? This person can become sick for life or die sooner than expected.

This diet maker claims that he is not a calories counter nor a protein pro. But almost 90 percent of his foods are bad animal protein, full of saturated fat, processed meats, smoked meats, seafood scavengers, and improperly prepared recipes. Again be careful of diet makers who tell people what they want to hear such as people can prepare an entire nutritious meal in seven minutes because some people in the USA think that time is money and they don't want to take the appropriate time to cook their foods. Sometimes people want fast results and the easy way out or time for entertainment instead of cooking. Other times, people prefer easy recipes with all the yummy and sweet desserts like uncooked cakes, cupcakes, flans, pies with raw eggs, high fructose corn syrup, corn syrup, refined white sugarcane, bleached flour, saturated butter, hydrogenated and partially hydrogenated or trans fat vegetable oil, heavy cream, artificial sweeteners, lots of preservatives and chemicals, and bacteria-laden animal products as weight-reducing diets.

Example Number 1

This diet maker tells people who want to lose weight, stay healthy, and fight certain diseases to take a half pound of ground turkey, make a patty with salt and black pepper, put vegetable oil on a frying pan on a stove, turn to four hundred degrees Fahrenheit for five minutes, turn the patty to brown, and place it inside a burger bun with lettuce and tomato. How in the world can poultry like turkey need one hour per pound at a temperature of 375 degrees Fahrenheit baked in oven until it reaches 185 degrees as in a hot thermometer to be cooked per United States Health Department can be healthy for people in just five minutes? No meat can reach the proper cooking temperature in five minutes. The five-minute cooked meat can only reach the danger zone, which is forty-five to fifty degrees Fahrenheit in a hot thermometer. And the danger zone is where bacteria multiply rapidly, especially salmonella in poultry.

Turkey, like all poultry, contain salmonella plus other organisms that need to be deactivated or put to sleep with time and temperature. Anyone in the United States who read labels or my previous book and is around me should know that by now.

True Story

One of my good friends and colleagues who told me about this diet book to buy and follow this diet almost lost her life. Let me tell you what happened to my friend and coworker, who swears by the goodness of this diet creator. She was a tall, slim, and nicely shaped blonde who just turned a forty-year-old divorcee. She wanted to maintain her figure so that she can start dating.

She bought that best-seller diet book and used it fervently to become a pro about foods, detailing the food composition of my diet, pointing out the benefits of each food in my plate, which was true. She said brown rice and dry beans, a lot of fibers; mixed vegetables of five different kinds vegetables in one meal and baked chicken, good protein; a Fuji apple with skin as dessert, low in calories, but rich in fiber; and eight ounces of spring water premeasured in a cup. "Hmm, that's great. You probably go to the bathroom many times a day. How many times?" I answered, "Three to four times a day depending on how many times I eat food rich in fiber." And she said, "Wow!" After listening to me for a while, she said, "You know about good foods. I want to know more about your wellness program, but my diet program is good too. Have you ever heard about the —— diet? You should buy the book."

Right after talking to me, she went to the kitchen in the workplace and made herself a plate of poison (according to the health department), sat by me, and ate with bare hands. That was the last time I saw her as a healthy, peppy, happy, and pretty lady. She disappeared for six weeks, and when I asked for her, thinking that she was in vacation, someone told me, "You don't know, Marie? She is very sick, can't even get up and out of bed. She has diarrhea, she goes to the bathroom five to fifteen times a day. She has blood in her stools for about six weeks besides high fever from infection and dehydration. She has twenty-four-hour nursing services at home, and we can only pray for her. Marie, she was thin already and now she's like a skeleton. On top of that, she's smoking and coughing." I said to myself, "Oh no, this butcher with his blank diet book is killing my friend."

When she finally scrambled herself out of bed and showed up at work, I didn't recognize her. She lost twenty-five pounds, which she didn't need to lose. She lost four dress sizes, and her face looked like a pack of bones. I could wrap around her waistline with both of my hands and make the thumbs meet. She said, "I know, Marie. I am miraculously alive. The doctor says that I need to gain fifteen pounds in a hurry." I opened my bag and gave her a cup of tea of my own composition. Before drinking it, she said, "Am I going to have diarrhea again from that tea?" I said, "No, honey, this tea is going to stop the diarrhea by clearing the poison out of your system. This poison is from the foods that this diet writer in this book told you to prepare in five minutes." I also told her that I would bring her a DVD of one of my presentations about foods good and bad. She said, "Oh, thank you, Marie." I did bring her the DVD. But that was the last time I saw that lady. I heard that she is doing okay, and now that I had published my first book, I plan on visiting her at the workplace to bring her my first book and later on this second book too.

Why I Brought Tea of My Own Composition at Work

I brought tea of my own composition at work for myself and sometimes for all the sick employees, which was about 85 percent after the holiday season. Many units were closed, patients were transferred to the hospital emergency room, and some employees were staying at home for some time. What I did at that time was call all the employees sick at home and tell a family member to shop for the needed ingredients to make their own remedy and come to work. All of them listened to me and did what I told them to do and came to work. All the employees who were sick at home called me or came to see me in person in my office when they signed their late slips or inquired about their work assignments. "I feel fine and energetic. What a good remedy you told my husband to make for me, I am now ready to work," one lady said to me. Unfortunately for me and these employees who were sick, that was my last time working at that place because one of my colleagues who had the same position as me told me, "You don't have to come here anymore, we will call you when we need you." I asked to see the big boss who was not there; I wanted to talk to the big boss over the phone. The same lady told me, "I talked to her already and she is not at home now."

Her story was this: She worked in that place for twenty-five years and couldn't find employees to cover all the units in that place that was full of old sick people for several shifts. Even after she bribed them as usual, they were too sick to get out of bed. When I got the employees' telephone book, she said to me, "I called them already, Marie, and they are all too sick to come to work even for me." I said to her it doesn't matter; after I talk to them, they all are going to be well enough to come to work. She said, "It's already after 11:00 PM and the shift has started. How can they get well enough to make it before this shift ended and the other shift started?" "Watch me and you will see," I said to her. Some of these people couldn't even come to the phone to talk to me because they were shivering, their teeth chattering with high fever, cold sweat, and them being wrapped up with several blankets. They were sneezing, coughing, cramping, and having diarrhea. I said to whoever I talked to over the phone, "Believe and trust for once in your life." They did exactly what I told them to do for their loved ones and gave them to drink a tea of my own composition, which sent the flu virus or bacteria toxin causing those people sickness from the holiday food parties straight to hell.

Although this coworker was happy to find people to work, her feelings of jealousy and insecurity were stronger than the temporary happiness. I also saved her life too because she was coughing, sneezing, shivering, having mucus running down her nose from the same party foods and I gave her the rest of my tea and left nothing for myself. After that day, I was never called to return to work in that place. I didn't call either to find out what went wrong. After that evening, a lot of coworkers called me to inquire about my absence. I told them that I was told to come back to work when I got a call from that person. I waited for a call to go back to work that never came. For several years now, I stay home and work on my books and my program T.H.A.T.S. and stay healthy.

Food Poisoning

To complete that segment with all the sick people in that place I worked some time ago, I'd like to say that it was not just me who helped my friends and coworkers to get better. What did it is my knowledge of food protection and infection control. If you refer to book number 1 T.H.A.T.S., The Health Assistance to Some, *you will know about food protection and infection control in depth too just like me.*

Most of the time, especially after the holiday seasons, a lot of people contracted food poisoning and think that they have a flu virus, stomach virus, or a bad cold. All I did was identify the possibility and composed a mixture of regular tea, ginger root, cinnamon stick, and lemon juice and told those sick people to first breathe it and drink it next steaming hot to wash out the toxin from the leftover party food. And bingo, that was the probability that I expected.

When it comes to health, the doctors, the hospitals, the pharmaceuticals, the nurses, the nursing homes, the dietitians, the nutritionists, and the pills are there for them in case of food poisoning or other conditions. That is what most people think. But I say prevention with knowledge is the best. Some people go to the gym every day, exercise, look fit, look in shape and not fat at all with nice and lean muscles, but never eat a home-cooked meal. I know some people who never use their kitchen or never even rent an apartment with a kitchen and spend a big part of their life eating out in restaurants, food trucks, food machines, takeout, and street-food carts. Although they look good physically on the outside, inside, their arteries are clogged. And their blood is as thick as maple syrup. One day any without sign, symptom, or warning, they will just collapse, have a heart attack, stroke, a diabetic shock or go into a coma, and die.

To me, no matter what people do to keep healthy, if they don't eat good, nutritious, organic, all-natural, protected food cooked at home, they are going to pay for that by collapsing at work, on their way home, in the gym, and on the streets. Because there is nothing that can replace good food. And no matter what anyone can tell me, good food can only be cooked at home by someone knowledgeable of food protection and infection control, which are both in the first book T.H.A.T.S. *If you don't have it yet, purchase it at the following Web site: Mariethats.com before you finish reading this book.*

The Ideal Restaurant

My husband and I talk about the only way that the restaurants could have served protected foods is by charging tremendous amount of money for their meals. And we wouldn't mind paying for that and eating out more often without fear of food poisoning. The question is why. And the answer is because the owners would have to hire educated people to only even clean the place. The owner would have to do the following: Starting with the building itself, the owner would have to build or remodel the building according to some health department's codes for the plumbing, the sewer system, the layout of the restrooms, the kitchen, the ceiling, the electrical fixtures, and the lighting.

The owners would have to open an accredited food protection school in place and make sure that they teach and train their employees food protection and infection control. For the employees to be qualified, they should have at least a BS degree in science, for example, physics, chemistry, biology, microbiology, nutrition, and culinary arts. To me, a BS will do, but master's is preferred.

The owners should have health-department nonbiased food inspectors in place or their own 24-7 supervisors keeping an eye on the place and employees at all time, making sure that they know and follow food protection and infection control at all times so that all rules and regulations and codes are enforced at all times. They should make sure that the trucks that carry the foods are refrigerated at a temperature of twenty-eight to forty degrees Fahrenheit at the most. And the food should not take more than twenty minutes to load and unload from the trucks to the restaurant's refrigerator and freezer.

The restaurant owners should make sure of where the employees live, whether they take showers every day, shampoo, shave, brush and floss their healthy teeth, apply unscented clear deodorant before wearing clean clothes, cut their nails short and keep them clean every day, comb their hair and pin them up, and wash their hands with warm water and liquid soap and dry them before they leave home for work.

The restaurant owners should have their own doctors with their own laboratories and graduated technicians to check the employees' health and make sure that the employees never come to work while sick. And before leaving home to come to work, the employees should not have a sore anywhere on their body nor a cold and especially hepatitis A, B, and C, and TB.

At work, all employees should pass an inspection before starting to work. Employees should wear uniforms, preferably white, a jacket or a lab coat, their hair pulled to the back and on top of the head, covered with a hairnet, a cap, or a hat.

Sinks with hot/cold water with good pressure should be accessible and available for hand washing with unscented regular soft liquid soap (non-antibacterial) in an automatic dispenser and plain white paper towel from an automatic dispenser to dry hands (no electrical air dryer please) at every six feet parameter. The entire place should be spotless, very clean, sanitized and dry, but no smell of deodorant, perfume, or any scent at any time that can cover the bacterial smell.

Cleaning and food preparation equipment should be obvious, exposed for everyone to see them. And knives, pots, spatulas, spoons, etc., that handle raw food should never be used to handle cooked foods nor different types of foods. If these rules are not enforced, the owners for sure would have to deal with cross contamination from germs multiplying in the foods by fifteen minutes at first then by twenty to thirty minutes from two to three bacteria to a million by one hour and keep on multiplying.

The employees should not smoke, chew tobacco, or drink alcohol. They should not be fat or obese because it could be harder for them to stay clean and dry by not sweating in a hot environment. Employees should wash and dry hands after eating, drinking, touching hair and clothes. Employees should never comb their hair, wear makeup, cut their nails, and rub their hands together for twenty to thirty seconds while at work. Employees should never taste food with their hands and put spoons or forks back to the pots after tasting. Employees should use a saucer to taste foods. Employees should never touch raw foods and then cooked foods without washing their hands and donning gloves to prevent cross contamination. As a matter of fact, to quote one of my professors, Dr. Herman Berkowitz, on Monday, March 25, 1996, at the Health Department Food Protection Academy, he said, "To prepare foods, wear disposable gloves, to handle foods be very careful and try very hard to handle foods as little as possible. Avoid hand contact, avoid cross contamination." He also said that gloves should never be an excuse for not washing hands; hand washing should never be an excuse for not wearing gloves. Gloves should be changed between touching different types of food, cooked and raw. Touching chicken and turkey full of salmonella and touching bread, salad, vegetables, fruits, and steak with the same gloves is a NO-NO. *The same professor also said that foods should never be touched (cooked or raw) with bare hands. People need something between their hands and foods. This something is called barrier in food protection and infection control. For this knowledge, refer to the book* T.H.A.T.S., The Health Assistance to Some, *at mariethats.com.*

OTHER DANGEROUS ORGANISMS

Virus

The fastest and direct way to contract virus is from our hands touching foods and utensils that we use to prepare and handle foods. Other ways are touching our noses, mouths, eyes; sneezing; blowing our noses; spitting in a thin tissue and holding it in our hands; and last, coughing and talking while dealing with foods and also being in contact with someone else. That is the way we usually contract viruses. Some are deadly and others are not. Sometimes we contract viruses coming from our hands and body cavities, including pores and body fluids. Although all diseases contracted from viruses are dangerous, some are more predominant in restaurants, for example, hepatitis. With all these different types of hepatitis, one would be foolish to deal with each other and with their foods without using barriers and protection.

What We Know about Virus

According to the U.S. Food Protection Program from the Health Department, we do not know too much about virus. We know a lot about bacteria, which I talked about in my previous book T.H.A.T.S. (The Health Assistance to Some). *We know food illnesses, biological hazards, how to see bacteria, what they look like, their two states, what they like and what they don't like, what can stop them from growing and multiplying. There are two ways that bacteria can make us sick: (1) by eating the live or dead bacteria and (2) by eating their waste or toxin or intoxication.*

Furthermore, we know that viruses don't grow on food. They grow on people. And people transfer them to foods. Viruses are very small, one hundred times smaller than bacteria. They grow by the day. In a city of Ohio, there was the Norwalk virus. We know that there is the rotavirus, cold virus, pneumonia, HIV, a few hepatitis viruses, stomach virus, and the flu virus. And now we have the swine flu or H1N1 flu virus. Since we know that virus don't grow on foods but on people, so to protect our foods and each other from viruses, we need to prevent direct contact with our food cooked and raw and each other. In the chapter of diseases and cure, I will talk in great detail about some illnesses contracted from virus.

In my previous book, T.H.A.T.S., *I explained a lot about bacteria, mold, and fungi. In this book besides virus, I will explain a little about parasites. Health departments know a lot about parasites, and from them, I know a lot too. But since they are not that important about disease-causing organisms, I will talk only about the ones that we have the most in our foods that can harm us.*

Parasite

According to the Health Department, all pork products are assumed infected, pork that look grayish in color, have cysts in the stratified muscles that can cause pain, muscle ache, chill, fever, flu. Trichinoses travel through the body, eyes, muscles, and diaphragm. The worms in fish cause a disease called anisakiasis.

KNOWLEDGE OF GOOD FOODS

I like to read anything about foods good or bad no matter where the reading comes from. Sometimes people make fun of me for reading tabloids because they think that they are not a good source of knowledge. These people don't know that knowledge is knowledge and is good or bad no matter where it comes from. It is up to the readers to know better, to assort them and pick up what is valuable to them and their loved ones. And I am sure that after reading T.H.A.T.S. or this book, the readers are going to be smart and knowledgeable enough to pick up the good knowledge and advice and reject the bad knowledge and advice about foods. Pay attention and see for yourself what I read in a magazine from someone giving advice about good deals that are bad to avoid. Some of them are good advices, for example, clipping coupons and buying seasonal fruits and vegetables. But some others about foods are really bad, and you shouldn't take these types of advice now that you have the power of knowledge about food protection.

This is a direct quote from the adviser: "Cooking meals from scratch isn't always a less expensive alternative to ready-made dishes. If the recipe calls for lots of ingredients, out-of-season items, or expensive foods, it's no money saver. Consider a baked or roasted entrée from your grocer's deli department." For health's sake, please don't do it! If you can cook your meals from scratch by following recipes that call for lots of ingredients in or out of season, more power to you! I compliment your intelligence, aptitude, and bravery for saving your health and your loved ones. Why in the world would you rather save money instead of lives, your own and others? And how do you know if you really saved money by buying these ready-made baked goods from the grocer's deli? With all the listeria, campylobacters, salmonella, bacillus Cereus, and E. coli you are bringing home with you to eat, who knows how much money you could have spent in health care if you take that advice?

According to my several decades of living in this country, studying, reading statistics and researching, to me and other researchers, American people compared to other countries rich or poor spend less money in food than the others. American people and America are among the richest people and the richest country, spending the biggest money on material stuff and junk, but the cheapest spender in foods. They are always looking in circular for food bargain, food on sale, reduced foods, food coupons, outdated foods, disintegrated foods, and artificial foods. And the newest trade now is auction food by large bulk that can give them a few months of supply. How in the world did these people come with that idea of auction for foods and buying food that can last that long? If anyone told me, I wouldn't believe it. But I got to watch it in the news on TV. Among these foods from a big carton was a leg of cow not on ice that was to last for three months too.

Another very interesting subject that I notice is a new addition to the chemicals and additives to foods to make them last even longer. I am not going to name them by the actual names given to them because so far, no other writer has noticed nor talked about them. What I am going to do is tell you about the element in them, which are alcohol, benzene, and aluminum, which have no place in food as safe additives. They are in our foods to make them last longer so that the companies wouldn't throw away the rotten foods and lose a profit. They don't care about how many people die per year with so many diseases, new types of bacteria, cancers, viruses, new types of flu, for example, swine flu. Please, people, open your eyes and read what is in your foods to make them last from three months to two years. Ask yourselves this: Since when do foods last that long and still be good food? Anything that last that long from the farm, the tree, the industry, the box, the can, and the package can't be 100 percent food anymore. They may look like food, taste like food, but can be poison and cause you harm. A lot of the food industries put their greed before people. Don't put your greed to cause diseases on some poor innocent people that can't fight back. People, don't buy anything called foods that can last that long on the grocery store shelves to save money or for the food companies to make money. This process is there for one purpose, the greedy people who's saving, making and accumulating billions of dollars of people with their long-lasting food garbage. I feel so sorry and heartsick to see some people buying their garbage as foods.

I watch in the news on TV a lady talking about saving money in food shopping while she was just dropping the packs of meat and poultry in the shopping cart without looking at them for color, liquid running in the package, expiration date, USDA sign, inspection's fact, handling instructions, cooking time, storage facts, and temperature and storage duration and where. My husband said to me, "Honey, look what this lady is doing. She is dropping these packs of meat and poultry in her shopping cart without looking at them, smelling them, turning them around for liquid and reading instruction, signs, content, etc." I answered him, "Well, she doesn't know and the reporter doesn't know either." They're not going to know unless someone tells them or if they read my book T.H.A.T.S.

In America at present or in 2008, there is another type of food store called Food Salvage. Some people might ask, what is that? Food salvage is a store that collect food from closed-out stores or foods that are unacceptable for normal or regular health-department-approved food stores. In these stores, you can buy a shopping cart full of foods that could have cost you approximately $250 from regular store, but cost you only $50 in the food salvage stores. Why? Because they have outdated, unsealed, unmarked, no-label, broken, and squashed cereal and pasta boxes; unwrapped animal products; broken, busted, and lopsided cans; and leaky jars and cellophane packages where air can go in. These foods can easily be contaminated and poisonous to people due to virus, parasites, and bacteria. It's in the media, in TV news for people to know. But people still buy them. For what? To save money and for the store owner to make money. At what risk? People's life and health!

Almost every day, I go to the supermarket to buy good foods for my family and also to help people buy these good foods too. Unfortunately, almost none of these people I want to help buy these good foods. When they held these bad foods in their hands and were ready to buy them, I told them, "No, buy these foods instead." They would answer back, "I can't afford it, they are too expensive." "Sir, don't you see what's in these foods?" He would answer, "Don't you see the price?" "But, sir, don't you see? Look at the color of your chicken, can't you smell the foul odor and see the liquid running in the package?" He said to me, "Oh, I buy it all the time like this. It's going to be cooked, and the bacteria will die." "Sir, if the bacteria will die, why will you need to put your food in the refrigerator after cooking it?" "I guess it makes sense, but we all are going to die of something." I said to this man, "Please take this chicken instead. Here's the money to pay for it, and don't ever feed your family and yourself with this type of foods again." When the foods look like that, they are bad for your health.

Another example, the same day, before I went to the register to pay for my foods, I met another man buying bread that was on sale and could last for six months in a big pack of twelve large pita breads. I walked to the bread, took a pack, and began to read it. I said, "Sir, why are you buying this bread? Look what are in it." He answered, "I know this is some kind of preservatives to make it last longer so the company wouldn't lose money." "So you know that the bread is bad and is made for the only purpose to make money and for you to save money because it's very cheap and you still buy it. So your only purpose is to get full and to save money." He answered, "Yes, we all are going to die one way or the other." This is unbelievable. Some people in the United States are driven by greed of either to make money or save money and forget about saving their lives and others. I don't know how crazy is that, but I had seen some billionaires eating foods that look like garbage on TV shows. Either they don't know or they like to eat free foods. In reality, they were eating garbage because these foods were no longer foods.

Some people are really poor and can't afford to buy good foods but just eat to survive. For these people, I feel really bad and sometimes guilty for having good foods to eat with my family. But for some rich and greedy people who are making money and saving money by eating and selling bad foods, I hope they realize their mistakes sooner or later and stop.

Honestly, not all the examples are bad, and not all the people I tried to help are not receptive and pessimistic as in the two examples before. I remembered helping a lady with a shopping cart full of junk foods by asking her to put back all the foods in her cart and let me choose healthy foods for her. I also told her why while doing it with her. This is how it went. She had juices with 5 percent juice and the rest with water and high-fructose corn syrup and corn syrup. She had cakes, cookies, candies, all with high-fructose corn syrup and refined sugar, refined bleached flour, potato chips, corn chips, salted pretzels, fatty cheese, cereal without fiber and with high-fructose corn syrup, and red shiny and rotten apples full of wax. She had some smoked salted meats and cold cuts. When I told her "These foods are not good for your health," she said, "I know, but my teenage daughter likes them. And all the foods now contain this high-fructose corn syrup. What can I do?" I took her to the aisles where they have naturally sweetened 100 percent juice next to the all-natural and organic cereals, pastas, snacks with seven whole grains, organic apples, other fruits, vegetables, salad, fresh poultry with reputable brand names after showing her how to examine them. Then we moved to the dairy aisle for fat-free and reduced-fat cheese, yogurts, milk, and eggs. And we went to the deli department where we got cold cuts in boxes with low sodium and fewer preservatives.

After we got a shopping cart full of good foods, she said, "Marie, you are an angel. I love you and will pray for you. You save me because I never know that you can find good foods in the same stores where there are bad foods. Knowledge is power, and we have to search, read labels, examine, and protect our foods and ourselves. Thank you, Marie." I said, "No problem, if you have any questions or problems, here is my phone number. Just give me a call and I will be there to help you."

Another time, my husband and I were shopping in a supermarket for produce. A nice lady approached us and said, "I have been observing you picking your vegetables especially the green beans, and I wonder why you take so long and be so careful with the beans." We explained to her that she had to look for insect bites, firmness, and the darkest and liveliest beans. We helped her with other green vegetables and sweet potatoes for her daughter. We exchanged phone numbers, and one day she called to say thank you. We recognized her right away and were pleased to help her at any time she needed us.

There is another moneymaker by using plastic bottles for almost everything, even for baby's bottles. What happened to glass bottles? Other countries rich or poor are still using glass bottles for food jars and drinking bottles for everything, including water, juices, and especially baby's bottles. Even though people in America know that some plastic can make people sick, they are still using them. Some industries know that the chemicals in these bottles can make people sick and yet force them on people who don't know or don't have a choice. Saving time to make money, saving money by using chemicals and poor-quality foods, and buying and eating cheap, reduced, and contaminated foods is not a wise practice at all.

The best way to solve some health problems is to take time to know about foods good or bad, to shop for good foods, to eat a rich diet of good foods, safe and nutritious and fresh foods. Shop at least every other day for good foods. And eat foods the same day or the most in three days after shopping and cooking them. Refer to T.H.A.T.S. (The Health Assistance to Some) book to know about food protection and good and bad foods.

According to statistics, people in America in 1968 used to spend 18 percent of their salary in food. Foods were not so expensive, but were good, organic, and natural. And people were healthier, slimmer, fit, and more energetic and more peaceful. And we had less billionaires than now in 2008. The statistics now in 2008 says that people make more money and spend less than 10 percent on food annually. Some average families spend on average $500 a year on food. To me, this is unbelievable. Last Sunday night, I was sitting in my parked car waiting for my husband. It was the garbage pickup the next day for a rich neighborhood in Brooklyn, New York. While there, I observed people looking in the garbage cans and wondered what they were looking for. Then I noticed that they were looking in the white plastic bags for beer cans and the black plastic bags that lined the garbage can for foods. I asked myself how can some people in a rich place like this be so poor to have to eat from a garbage can.

But I found out the next day on the news of channel 7 ABC that people look in the garbage for foods just to save money, rich or poor. I also saw a lady being interviewed by a reporter who picked a black garbage bag by the sidewalk that contains bagels when she opened it. She tasted a bagel and let the reporter taste one also. I couldn't believe it! The lady told the reporter that these bagels were from the previous day. But to me, even if they were from the previous day, it doesn't mean that they are safe to eat for many reasons: Since they were discarded as old products, they probably were treated as garbage, which was on the bare floor. Or people working there probably walked on them with their street shoes after walking in dog's excrement, vomit, green infected, contaminated mucus with all kinds of bacteria and viruses. The garbage bag made for garbage may contain fiberglass, asbestos, and other chemicals, which are not good for eatable foods. Eating in garbage is a very risky and life-threatening business. To me, these people who are saving money are destroying their lives. No wonder in the United States we have so many people with so many types of cancer, so many new diseases, obesity, and diabetes as pandemic.

THE CHEMICALS

Remember the chemicals I told you that were contained in the foods that the gentlemen were buying? Here they are: some margarine that contain partially hydrogenated oil, vegetable or soybean oil, hydrogenated cottonseed oil, whey in milk are bad.

Salt (table salt) or Sodium (not too bad)
Vegetable oil with trans fat (bad)
Mono and triglycerides (bad)
Soy lecithin (not too bad)
Potassium sorbate (good)
Calcium disodium EDTA to protect quality (not too bad)
Citric acid (good)
Artificial flavor made with other foods (good)
Vitamin A (good)
Palmitate (not too bad)
Beta-carotene color, beets color (good)

All bad additives are the following:

Dextrose
Corn sugar
Corn syrup
High-fructose corn syrup
Inverted sugar
Maltitol
Mannitol
Polydextrose
Salt or sodium chloride (use only from 0–2 percent in products)
Sorbitol
Sugar or sucrose
Xylitol

Artificial colorings are the following:

Citrus red 2, red 40
Brominated vegetable oil

Butylated hydroxyltoluene
Quinine
Artificial coloring yellow 5

There are more of the bad chemicals, but I can only name some in this book. You can refer to the previous book T.H.A.T.S. *for more chemicals and additives that are good, not too bad, and bad.*

Before I move to the next chapter, which is about diseases and foods to help or cure them, I want to introduce you, readers, to this chapter called wisdom.

WISDOM

Wisdom is included in this book because to me, it's part of healthy living. It makes you think before you act. It also makes you realize that every action you take has a reaction. If the reaction is a good surprise, you learn something good. But if it is something bad that you learn, you know that you made a mistake and that you have to take responsibility to correct it. Therefore, to me, wisdom is a part of our lives in order for us to be healthy.

Wisdom, according to my philosophy, is what follows:

Don't leave for later or tomorrow what you can do now or today.

Don't do anything without a plan and a purpose.

Don't do anything without preparation; even a little prep is better than none.

Even when you improvise or are in an emergency, take a few seconds to think of what to say or do.

Instead of being selfish, be selfless. Be kind, compassionate, and generous to other people too, not just to yourself all the time. Even in an emergency, be calm and composed, chill out, but don't waste time or energy needlessly.

Be humble. It cost nothing to be humble, and smile to other people and say hi. Be happy with one another, take a day of the week for enjoying with loved ones, and play table games or have picnics outside with family, friends, and loved ones instead of running to work all the time or somewhere else.

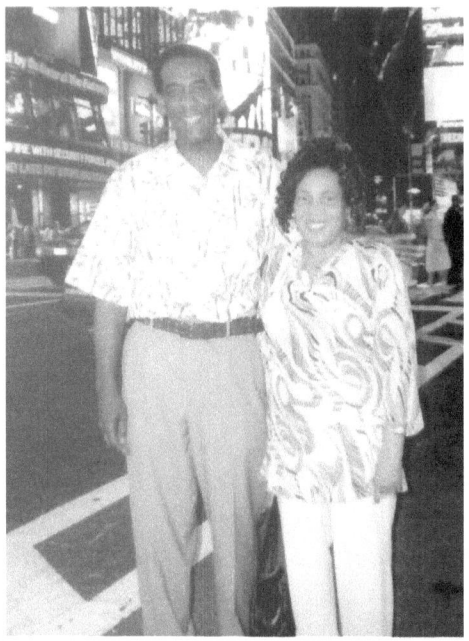

"My husband Eddie and I chilling out in New York City at Times Square"

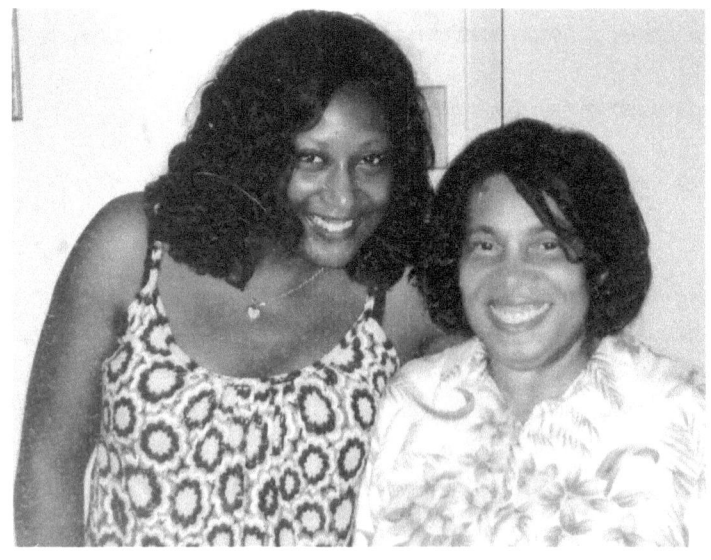

"Enjoying a summer visit at my daughter Karen's house"

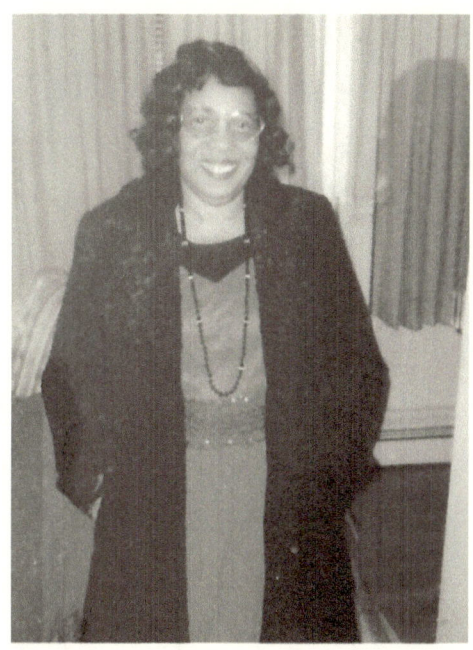

"Winter holiday at my daughter Karen's house"

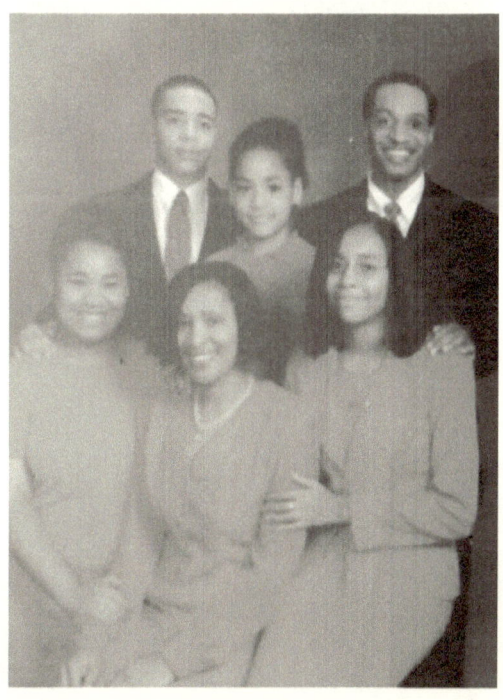

"My oldest son Rico's family"

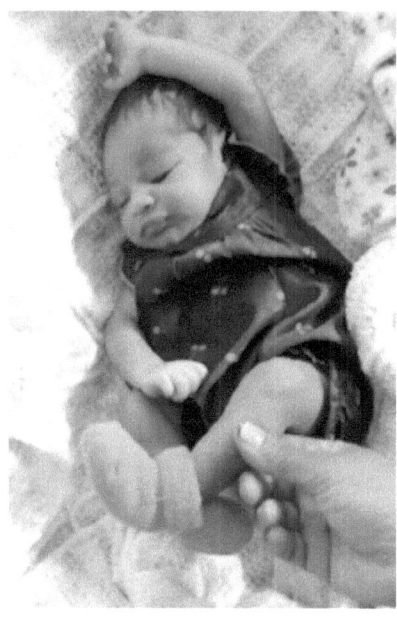

"Baby girl Sydney, the latest addition to the family"

Good thinking for good health starts with enjoying your life and watching other people enjoy their life.

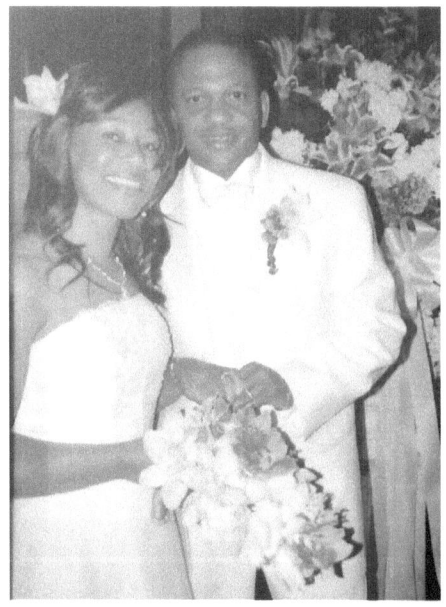

"My nephew Patrick and his wife on their wedding day"

Keep out negativity. Don't become recluses who don't go anywhere because some people enjoy talking so negatively about others behind their backs and because you don't like that. Just don't take part of it. It's okay to socialize.

Don't be cruel. Sometimes while watching TV you can cry or feel bad when you see people being cruel to each other and some poor innocent children or animals and for destroying earth with garbage that is making us sick.

I love people, animals, and the planet Earth at the time that we are living on it.

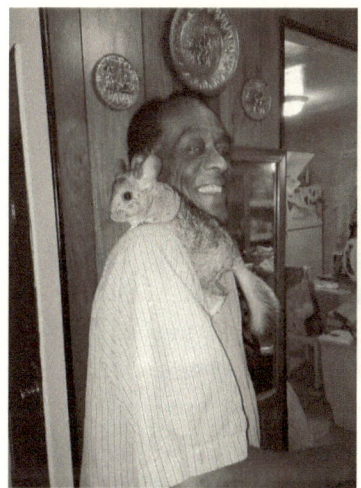 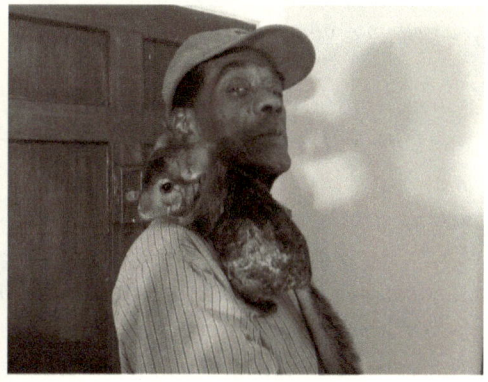

"This is my husband Edouard holding our male chinchilla named Melvin and our female chinchilla named Joana"

Know to set priorities and don't pass up opportunities because you might not get them again.

Do or say what you know first if possible before you say anything else. If not, go with your heart and then your head or gut feelings.

Often seek knowledge, education, learning, and help because these make you who you are.

Don't think that you know enough, too much, or don't need to know or need the help.

To me, knowledge is vital and not just power. When it comes to knowledge, think of it as the sky is the limit.

Don't lose opportunity to learn, to acquire knowledge, and to educate yourself.

Share your knowledge with others, whether they want it or not. Just know that they can benefit from it and you give it to them free of charge sometimes. Help people understand the knowledge so they can pass it around to others.

There are times that you might go down. But if you go down, don't let yourself go down too far and for too long.

If that happens, pick up yourself first by giving thanks to the Almighty for your faith on life and the next for whatever is left for you because no matter what happens, it could have been worse. Cheer up and entertain yourself, pick up a tabloid, and read a farfetched story; or if you are too low and can't even read, just look at the silly pictures and laugh. Think of something hilarious but happy that happened in the past and smile wide, even talk to yourself and say how ridiculous that was and laugh again even louder. I am 100 percent sure that you will feel better right away, now already. Don't say I will be okay later. You are fine now as long as you are still breathing. Do you want to know why? Because laughing produces feel-good hormones from your body so that you can see your way out from the low condition that you are in. You can have a clear mind, energy, initiative to make plans, to have dreams, promises to yourself and goals that you can fulfill. And not only will you be successful but your success can also be beyond your expectations and your imagination.

Whatever you have to do, don't say it's too hard or I can't do it before you even try it.

Try it and try it again, remember to change approach at each trial until you get it. Plan it, make a schedule, practice it, rehearse it, and picture it in your mind. And you will get it sooner than you think. Whatever you want to do or to get, just work hard for it.

Don't go for easy because easy is just easy; it doesn't mean that it's good. Just remember that easy can more likely be bad.

Go for good or the best no matter how hard it is. Do not be too content and stop there. Keep moving, and don't be stagnant because everything is moving forward. Therefore, say to yourself, "That's good, but it could have been better. I will try to do better next time, or faster and cleaner." But keep your promise. There will be a next time unless you already reach the top and there is no other way to go but the other side.

In almost every task you perform, go for excellence and move on to the next.

Almost every job, assignment, or task that you have to perform, to do, or to create, say to yourself, "I don't just like this job and my boss, I love both of them." And guess what? Since you already psych yourself, no matter how bad both of them are, it becomes real for you because it's mind over matter.

Often do your job with care, a smile, a conscience, and close to 100 percent of your ability.

No matter what it is that you are doing for a living, make sure that you know about it and give it your best.

Don't work for pay alone. No no! Work for self-worth, enjoyment, socialization, for meeting or being around people, learning, being active, exercising, practicing self-growth and development, and for the benefit of your employer and humanity. If it is for yourself, do the same above and take pride in what you do. Consider the pay or the profit as an icing on the cake to make a living.

Wherever you are and whatever you do and however you feel inside, know that it is yours only and is private. Just know that being sad, angry, grouchy, and crabby will not solve your problems and that the people around you or meet are not responsible. Therefore in a work environment or elsewhere, be always happy on the outside, smile wide, be courteous and caring for others; it will be enough to make whatever you feel inside lose all power over you. Your positive attitude, your happiness, and your big smile will become real for you and others. And suddenly, the problems and bad feelings you had before will be all over and turn to great solutions and joy.

Do not fight feelings and emotions. Just replace them with each other. Remember, there is a positive for every negative. And only you know your feelings. To name some:

sadness	happiness
selfish	generous
down	up
violent	peaceful
hate	love
dislike	like
angry	glad
taking	giving
mad	serene
frowning	smiling
grimacing	laughing
grouchy	joyful
indifferent	caring
greedy	sharing
vengeful	forgiving
arrogant	humble

The great news about replacing the bad and negative attributes with the good and positive ones is that they cost you nothing except a little effort. With knowledge and education, planning, self-discipline, organization, and hard work, you can accomplish a lot with some help and guidance.

Remember that it is healthier, faster, and better for anyone to love than to hate, to praise, to compliment, and to forgive than to criticize negatively, to hold grudges, to belittle, and to disrespect.

To quote Edgar Allan Poe, "To vilify a great man is the readiest way in which a little man can himself attain greatness."

It is bigger to apologize and accept your fault, your mistakes, and take responsibility than to deny, find excuses, and blame. Blaming each other is another thing that I can't take. Please stop blaming each other, stop telling people what to do, and stop driving other people crazy by giving them orders. Let young and old people be themselves for a change as long as they are not destructive to themselves and to others.

Almost always, feel that you are on a mission, that you are carrying a message that you have to do something good or pass it on to others. Even if you don't know what it is, try to be compassionate; do something good to someone or for someone; say hi, how are you; be courteous and respectful, and more good ideas about doing good things for people will come automatically. That act definitely will help you and others, and it's for free of charge.

Self-Help and Helping Each Other

Watch and see if people can help themselves and others in doing something positive and good. If in need, help them too. You can help them find jobs if they want to work, go to school for self-education, be an artist, play music, sing, decorate, garden, farm, play sports, read literature, cook, etc. Help and encourage people in anything else except that cell phone, which some people are being glued to all the time. It is a great invention, especially for communication and keeping us in touch with each other in any occasion, place, or time. But to me, people should use it with caution for their own good and others.

Even if someone does something for you for money or as your employee, say thank you, compliment the good, and if the bad is not that bad, forget it or overlook it or correct it yourself. If you have to make corrections, do it privately, don't let the person know about it, and don't pass it around to other people.

Don't confront and reprimand someone harshly. It's better to call the person in a private area and talk to him or her calmly.

Don't blame, accuse, condemn, instigate, and be the judge and the jury before you even know how something wrong happens to or is done by someone because you might find yourself in the same situation also and hope for someone nicer than you for help. And if really this someone did something wrong or made a mistake, don't say, "You are wrong! And this looks bad or terrible."

It's better to just say, "It is different from what I expect and thought. Let's see if and how we can fix it." Or you can say, I don't do it this way, there is another way that I like better. Remember, there is no one way to do everything. You might not know the other ways sometimes, but that doesn't mean that they are not there. The other ways can be better, worse, or have the same result as yours. And no one would know unless you try them. Remember, because of the brain, we have different levels of intelligence, perception, feeling, senses, and sensation. Although in some aspects we are unique, we all fall under some categories on the spectrum. Don't think that you are the most of anything because whatever you are the most, someone else is more than you. Whatever you do best, someone else can or has done it way better than you. When it comes to the spectrum, all you can hope for is to be placed in either one of the two extremes or in the middle where most people are. It's called the norm or normal, average, or standard. The reason is more people fall under this spot. And this people do almost the same thing the same ways almost all the time. But once someone is at either extreme, than tension is created, and this person is in constant trouble from the normal people, which are the majority. As a matter of fact, some people think that normal people are only the good and healthy people. And the people under the two extremes are sick and freak or supernatural.

When you are in the extreme above the norm, some people admire you at first, can't do without you, overuse you and want to be like you but can't. They next turn jealous, become angry at you, envy you, dislike you, try to destroy you, get sick around you, try to compete with you, lose control around you, plot to destroy you, go against you, find fault in you, negatively criticize you, watch your every move, despise you, and can't understand you. But one thing for sure that they can't do is they can't change you or even touch you. On the contrary, the more they persecute you, the more their plans against you will backfire. Why? Because you know them better than they know themselves. And you, just for being in the above extreme, you have qualities that prepare you for any event, which makes you several steps ahead of them. Rarely, they can trip you if you get distracted and lose your touch.

When you are at the extreme below the norm, you get humiliated, ridiculed, yelled at, screamed at, criticized negatively by the norm, pushed down, called names—for example, dumbbell, retarded—talked bad about you behind your back, have pity on you, have mercy on you, and feel embarrassed to be around you. At the below-norm extreme, to some people, you are their self-worth, self-confidence, and pride. The below-norm extreme are instrumental in increasing the norm's self-esteem and ego because the norm think that if the below norm can make it, they can make it too ten times more and better.

In conclusion, when you are in the above-norm extreme, you suffer the most while the norm and the below norm are rejoicing at your expense. If you pay attention, from their behavior, you can almost hear them saying, "Yes, you are so high up on your horse, you think that you know so much that you don't need them and you are so happy and content, we must give you some zappers so we can see who is laughing now." But guess what? You already know what they are capable of. And it doesn't bother you nor touch you one way or the other.

The above-norm extreme can continue to be there if they know themselves and what they want out of the position and not abuse it.

The below-norm extreme can learn, educate themselves, be patient, and ignore the norm sometimes and better themselves, can increase or upgrade their position to the above-norm extreme.

The norm is usually the one that get it made with less effort; because they are so sure of themselves, they turn to be the bullies. And most of the time, they get tolerated by other norms because they are the majority, the most popular, the most everything that sometimes they don't even try or think about going above. What more can they want since they are the norm and everything's good and healthy. For them, the two other extremes are the bad, the sick, and the unusual. Therefore, the norm are the people that make the statistics for everything too.

And sometimes after all the mistreatment, when you are gone and it's too late, that's the time that the norm, the above-norm extreme, and the below-norm extreme missed you and saw how good or even great you were, how much good things you did for some of them, and how low you were and brought yourself up and all the good qualities you fortunately had.

Knowing Where You Are

No matter where you are or if you don't know where you are, you can find out by doing the following:

Do a soul-searching and find yourself. And give yourself a quiz.

Ask yourself these questions:

Who am I?
What do I want?
What do I do best?
How long and how much can I do what I do best?
What do I really like or dislike?
How far can I go?
Am I in the right direction?
How do I see or perceive myself?
Where do I feel the most comfortable?
What are my dreams?
What are my priorities?

You can always ask yourself more questions since you should know yourself better than anyone.

When you finish your quiz, grade it and be honest to yourself and don't discriminate, don't deny, be fair, and don't beat yourself up for what you can't answer. It will come to you with practice.

Also, make yourself two lists. List number one with your strengths, what moves you up and forward. List number two is the one with your weaknesses, what holds you down or keep you stagnant and bring you back.

List number one is your strengths list or your good qualities.
List number two is your weaknesses and your bad qualities.

List number one enumerates all your strengths, your courage, your gifts, your talents, your heroism, your tenacity, your continuity, your following up with projects, your good dream, your creativity, your artistic ability, your wisdom, your integrity, your honesty and loyalty, your hard work, your motivation, your audacity, your willpower to survive, and your happiness. This is the list that keeps you up and moves you forward with positive attitude and laughter and endurance no matter what.

List number two is your weaknesses or all your detrimental and bad qualities that you might have. They are your lack of perseverance, your negative thinking, your ambivalence, your fear of taking risks, your lack of continuity, lack of following up, your lack of any amount of thrust to anything and anyone, your lack of activity, your lack of creativity, your lack of motivation, your promptness to give up, your impatience, your discouragement in tedious situation or work, indifference to others, lack of care, belligerence to learning, stopping others who want to progress, isolation, negative criticism, and other bad qualities that you know already that are not on this list.

From the list number two, eliminate the most of the bad qualities as soon as possible. And replace it with good qualities from list number one. That's why you have to start with the list number two first so you wouldn't have too much of them left.

Next, go to number one list and add some more good qualities. And take the ones you want the most and turn them to a dream, have a vision of it. And turn it to reality. Sometimes it can be more than one dream. In that case, set priorities and keep on trying and working at accomplishing your dream or dreams.

How You Work in Accomplishing Your Dreams

Start with your dreams one at a time or one by one.
Instead of making one plan as usual, make three plans:
Plan number one or A the best or the most wanted.
Plan number two or B, the next best thing.
Plan number three C, the acceptable or safety net.
Like this, you have the most confidence needed to accomplish your dream with plan A. Because you have options. You know for sure that your dream is coming true one way or the other. Therefore, you have no fear or less fear of overcoming bad surprises you may encounter in your way.

All your adrenaline, your good hormones, your enzymes and body juices can move you to the right direction with full strength through obstacles. Because if you fall, it will be into your safety net plan C after passing plan B, which is less likely.

Almost always we accomplished our plans with good planning strategy.

And if we start by ourselves and introduce others later on if needed, our plans can be carried to the letter and the result will be better than expected and even faster too. Another reason we have to include others later on is because we need to know some of our techniques and learn the plan ourselves before presenting it and explain it to others.

Know that the more people we have included to the plan, the less likely the plan will come true or be achieved. When we count on ourselves, the least likely we will let ourselves down. With the saying, "When push comes to shove" or when problems develop, we will be the only ones to stick to the plan and surely will not abandon the ship while the others will jump the boat. We are the captains of the boat or ship.

Team work is good, but sometimes we don't have the time to explain, to teach, to clarify and make others understand our plan too soon. Because not too many people have vision. And usually, what people can't see are more difficult for them to understand. It is better to start on our own until something is concrete for others to see, touch, feel, or hear. Then we can include others periodically because now, we have something to show and can understand and predict the rest of the plan and the outcome. Therefore, the plan becomes more possible.

In order to have visions, dreams, and plans, which we can execute and make real, we need to be at a certain level in the spectrum. Sorry to say it, but not all of us are in the same level. Remember at the beginning of this chapter, I mentioned the three levels: the below extreme, the normal, and the above extreme. There are also different positions or degrees of the extremes. People who are too much in the below normal can't even function. And people who are too far up in the upper extreme above normal don't last either because they are too controversial, unexplainable, daring, heroic, unbelievable, extraordinary, powerful, etc.

Although everyone needs a package, the package can't be too heavy.

On the contrary, if some people don't have a package or certain attributes, talents, gifts, intelligence, drive, qualities of the heart, emotion, spirits, or soul, things will just happen to them. Good or bad, they don't even know how to make them happen and how to benefit from the good and avoid the bad. These people might even let the opportunity go by and not grab it.

The people above average are usually so caught up or inclined or obsessed in what they are doing that they don't even take the time to relax, live their life fully, and rest. They work too hard in whatever they are doing and get themselves exhausted. Sometimes they get killed, kill themselves involuntarily, die as a martyr for a political or religious cause. Other times they die for science, inventions and experiments or just stressed themselves out by practicing some arts that they created.

Don't be alarmed if you are not too far down in the below-average extreme. With education, other knowledgeable people, professors, teachers, books, the media, and the Internet, you can acquire many good qualities or attributes that you were not born with. You can upgrade your IQ or intelligence by learning in schools, books, laboratories, experiments, experiences, and practices. Many people in our society who are educated and have many types of degrees from associate to doctorate are in the upper below average to average. And some others who are average and above in the upper extreme have no degrees at all. Meaning that it doesn't matter in what level some people are, they can acquire intelligence; improve their memory; increase their IQ; learn a trade, techniques, practice, experiment, experience; learn new behavior, lifestyle change, and how to protect themselves and their foods, which is in other chapters for diseases control.

Don't waste time and energy into details and miss the big picture.

Forget about controlling people, just try hard to control yourself and your situation.

Don't try to change people or their situations. To me, people can only change themselves and their situations. It is better to help other people change themselves and their situations for the better if they seek or want your help.

And hopefully, some troubled people who follow an example of good role model might be changed too.

If people really want to change for the better, they have to be honest, determined, work hard, have a positive attitude in life. And also, they have to be brave enough to take risks sometimes. To me, without risk, people get nothing. People who risk nothing get nothing.

People need to leave the comfort zone for the danger zone sometimes depending on the circumstances. Don't be too prompt on setting limits. People should not predict what they can do, how much they should do, how far can they go, or if they are willing to do that much or go that far and stop here or there. People need to be open-minded, broaden their horizon, be flexible, have an unknown limit, and keep going until they reach their goals or fulfill their dreams. Because no one really know these things. So why bother with predictions and expectations. Just have faith, patience, and hope for the best.

Avoid procrastination because no matter how hard and how long a job or task is, if people start it and do as little as possible at a time they can continuously, it will be finished someday and some time. People sight is the coward and not people. What that really means is your eyes see bigger than the job is.

Example Number 1

When children started the second grade of elementary school at age seven, they think that they will never finish and graduate. But they did and move on to high school. In high school, they say, "This is too much and too hard and we'll never make it." But they graduate and move on to college. The first day in college for their first degrees, they think four years is a long time. But they go anyway until graduation day. And then they say to themselves, "Oh boy, time passes fast. It wasn't that bad after all." They have their degrees and can get a better job. And for some of these people, if they really want, they can do it over and over. They just complete the requirements, have the knowledge, and forget about the graduations and the diplomas. They can just keep going and keep the promises to themselves to finish what they started and show to themselves how brave they are. They can go on to PhD, MD, doctoral, and postgraduate, internship, and have the career that they had been dreaming of or above and better than their plans or dreams. All people need is have faith, believe, and hope.

Some people are afraid to attend higher education classes until graduation. Others don't go to college or university at all for many reasons. Some go for a length of time and drop out along the way. Others stay until graduation, obtain a degree, run, and never go back. A few people stay and return for one, two, to three more degrees for higher positions and more money. But only a few people goes again and again just for the knowledge.

Upper Extreme above the Normal

When people are in the extreme upper above the norm, people admire them, can't do without them, follow them around, watch every move they make, like them, and want to be like them and make them their role model. Next they overuse them if they can, turn against them, become jealous, angry, dislike, and envy them for no apparent reason. Later on, they try to destroy them, get sick around them, compete with them, lose control around them, plot against them, find fault with them, blame them, negatively criticize them, watch every move they make, and despise them.

All the above happen because people don't understand the upper extreme above the normal. The normal are so used to people who act like themselves that they are the same as them, so they see red if these other people are different. But they can't change them, nor can't even touch them sometimes. On the contrary, the more the norm persecutes the extreme above, the more their plans backfire. Most of the time, the upper extreme know the norm better than they know themselves. If the upper extreme above the norm doesn't pay attention to the normal people or the norm, they can really get hurt sometimes. This time, I used "people" or "they" because some people may think that it's only them when I used "you" in the first description of the upper extreme above the norm. It's not just you, it's everybody in that place in the spectrum that goes through the process. That is why I repeat this segment, almost like the other that was previously stated.

Some of the people in the below-the-norm extreme can be living there unknown for a major part of their lives until they surprise everyone with their talents and gifts and climb instantly to the above-the-norm extreme one day.

For example, Susan Boyle at forty-eight years old became famous after her audition for a talent show while by looking at her and the way she described herself as a plain Jane who never really fit in can change. At school, she was hyperactive, cried easily, was bullied, was called Miss Piggy that no one and even herself would ever think that she will reach stardom and be worth several millions dollars at the present. How is that for gift, talent, and upgrading from lower extreme to upper extreme and bypassing the norm. I say wow!

Others in the above-the-norm extreme can make mistakes and blunders (according to the normal people) or norm. They can be tripped by the norm and fall flat on their faces. Sometimes, some above-norm or upper-extreme people get destroyed by the norm who dislikes them so much that they think their only solution is to get rid of them. Most of the time, the paparazzi, the politicians, the media, the comedians, the talk show hosts, and the photographers make a field day of the talented, gifted, the liberators, the entertainers or whatever these people have or can do that the norm don't have or can't do. Most of the time, these people in the upper extreme get very rich, go back to being very poor, get ridiculed, are verbally abused, suffer public injustice, die young in disgrace and alone. Sometimes it's only after their demise that all people recognize them.

Play Low-Key

In everything in life, there are some exceptions. For people in the upper extreme who are really smart, some things can be done for them so that they could live a long, happy, and peaceful life. These things are the following: They can play low-key, become a hermit, be undercover, and not advertise their millions of dollars and their talent. They can pick up a few honest, sincere, and loyal friends and family members whom they love and are still on their side and hibernate with them, get out of the fire right on time. The best way for them to get a break is to make everyone forget about them and run to the newcomers. They can start by playing low-key and slowly but surely get out of the limelight.

Just remember that in order to be in the above-norm extreme, most people have something that stand out like a thumb that everyone can see but can't explain and can't understand whether it's good or bad. The only difference is that they are the only people who have that something. That something makes them abnormal. The more something these people have, the more abnormal they become. And sometimes, the higher these people get, the lower, faster, and harder they fall. These people are also almost never predictable. Usually, no one knows what they are going to do next, even themselves, in a given situation.

People in the below-norm extreme are not so much different as the norm compared to the upper-norm extreme. Sometimes they can even pass as norm with minor difficulty. The norms stay longer in any situation. They climb to high positions and stay until retirement or the end of their lives. Most of the time, other people like them, love them, admire them. They continue what they started until the end. They are very predictable. They rarely change jobs, career, schools, residence, country, states, and even phone numbers. They do the same things at the same time, same age, and same ways sometimes at the same time. Sometimes, they have some minor discrepancies or differences, but not enough to be disqualified as the norm and not to be called anything else but the norm. And most of the time, the people at the norm expect others who are not in it to do the same things and like the same ways as them. If the other abnormal that they call them can't, don't know how, or refuse to do like them, they get punished, forced, or mistreated. To me, physically, emotionally, mentally, spiritually, and socially, the norm people are almost the same. No matter what they do, if they want to beat it, they can't. Rarely, some people in either extremes can get trapped in the norm. But they don't do well in there because the norm can smell them a mile away. They smell something fishy and really make it hard for them to stand. It's like if the norm is saying, "How dare you become one of us? Get out or we will destroy you or make you miserable!" "You are not like us, you are a fake." "We do things differently, we do things right, we get to places on time, and we mean business, we are organized, we have discipline, we are clean-cut, etc." What they don't say is "Except that we are average."

The people in both extremes who want to become norm are usually not happy, are persecuted until they recognize their place, who they are, and can say, "Who cares who you are!" "You are not good or bad. Just because you are the norm doesn't mean you are the best. Being the norm is a matter of numbers. You have the largest number, the greatest percentage, and the most same ways to do things or more popular, and that's it."

"People in both extremes, different than the norm, are who they are. They accept themselves, love themselves, and have a dream and work to attain it."

People should know that no matter where they are in the spectrum of society, they need to have integrity first to themselves and next to others in everything. And they should be brave too. People can have all the power, the money, the gift, the talent, the intelligence, and all the rest you name it; but if they don't have integrity, they can only be at the level that is next to the lowest in the spectrum. And if they are not yet there, they sure will be sooner or later. Know that all the good qualities in people are very rare. And a very few are almost impossible to find in our society. There are honesty, loyalty, caring, loving, compassion, humility, kindness, sharing, and real generosity. This generosity means that people shouldn't only give when they have too much or want tax deduction. It's when they have enough for themselves and give some of it to others who don't have at all; it's called generosity. Or they should give and not expect something in return.

This segment of the book is to help people know themselves and accept themselves for who they are, the way they are, and wherever they are in the spectrum of society. In order to be healthy, happy, and grateful for who they are, what they have and where they are in every sense of the word, people need to acknowledge these facts. I also have to clarify the word "norm" or "normal" in this segment because this word more likely means average in the spectrum of society. This norm or normal is not the same as for diseases and conditions or your medical test result.

My Beliefs

In order for people to be whole, complete, and healthy, they need to achieve homeostasis. People need to be emotionally, mentally, spiritually prepared before they can be physically healthy.

Although this book is mostly about physical health, we need to talk briefly about the mental, emotional, and spiritual health also because they interfere and interact with each other. They are parts of the whole in the equation. People can't be complete without all four healthy parts.

Spiritually Healthy

To be spiritually healthy, people need to believe in the universe, the infinite, the creation, themselves, and some percentage in others and some facts of life. I am not going in detail about this part of health. Why? Because each individual has his or her own definition of spirituality besides religion. What we need to do is a self-examination to know our beliefs and ourselves. I can give you a brief example of my beliefs or myself. It might not be what others believe of me.

Example Number 1

I believe that I am a hard worker, a determined person, and sometimes driven when it comes to seeking knowledge. I believe that I have perseverance, consistency, continuity, adherence to my plans and tasks until I achieve my goals.

I believe that I have a good positive perception and sensation about myself, other people, and events.

I believe that I am compassionate, patient, generous, honest, loyal, a good learner and teacher. And sometimes I can be tolerant because I love people.

I believe that sometimes I can be too conscientious, which makes me too hard on myself if some of my plans turned out differently than expected. If and when I make a mistake, I take it very hard. I take responsibility for my mistakes and correct them right away to the best of my ability. And if my mistakes involved others, I apologize and make it up to them.

Emotional Health

I believe that in emotional health, relationships play a big role. Let's talk about some relationships:

Children-Parents Relationship

I believe that parents should care for their children the best they could. They should love their children unconditionally. But they should set limits right away or as soon as possible. Otherwise, their children can get mixed messages.

Example Number 2

You as a parent want your child to stop doing something that you think is bad behavior. Just continue on the stopping regardless of what your child says or does and whatever psychological method you use as behavior modification. If you use time-out, or stand by the wall, no playtime, or no TV, etc., don't stop until your child stops the bad behavior completely. Immediately, teach your child good behavior that can replace the bad one and help him or her.

Know that all behaviors are learned and can be unlearned. In order to do that, you need to have continuity, consistency, and steadfastness in your rules and regulations. You need to have honesty, fairness, and not cave in. Do not use bribery or punishment. Do not give mixed messages. Remember that when you say no, it means no. You should never say no and yes after for the same behavior or request. Your no means only no and not sometimes yes. You can't say no sometimes and other times say yes to the same child or other children in the same family. Don't be afraid that your child or children don't like you or even don't love you as a parent. All the above can promote negative reinforcement and rebellion.

It is not about you; it's about your child or children's preparation for life. Be prepared to be disliked. Be able to make sacrifices. Know that your child or children are not a prize. They don't have to love you or like you to be good people later on. You as a parent have to love them unconditionally and let them know that as often as possible. You might not like what they do or who they become or who you will like them to be. But if they stay too long in that condition, it's not the time to change them. To me, it's too late. The manipulation, control, arguments, and the briberies are too late too. You can always try with no guarantee of success.

The right time was when they were very young and as early as possible. Because no one really knows when to start teaching children and when can children start learning. As far as scientific research, children can start learning from their mother's belly. What parents should do are the following:

1. *Draw a contract and make your child or children sign it.*
2. *Make them promise and keep their promises to stop what's wrong and start what's right as soon as you told them.*
3. *Make them acknowledge their wrongs and bad behavior and take responsibility.*
4. *Reward their good behavior.*
5. *Take away something they like until the bad behavior stops and is corrected and erased completely.*
6. *Don't worry if your child or some of your children don't like or don't love you. Just be grateful if they are alive and well and love them anyway.*
7. *Just remember that the wrong and the bad are easier to do than the good and the right. Also remember that you did what you believe was right and good for them.*
8. *Children don't come with a how-to-do manual. Parental psychology can help. But if you cannot have that knowledge on time, just remember that you did the best to your knowledge and have no regret. It's not just you! Most people in general including your child or children think that "the grass is greener on the other side."*
9. *Always respect your children, be honest with them; and when you are wrong, admit and apologize. Above all, provide autonomy and let him or her or them be their own self and not be an attachment or continuity to you as the parent.*
10. *Give trust, credit where it belongs, advice if requested, and privacy when needed.*
11. *Do not criticize negatively, do not provoke, do not blame. Be there for him or her or them and give support and encouragement when needed. Do not hold grudges. Do not give payback. Forget and forgive the bad and remember the good. Repeating the bad, punishing the bad, and giving payback are instant gratification due to the idea that does not last when the superego takes over. Remember, they are your loved ones. And when they hurt, you hurt too. Even when you are the one that hurts them.*

Work Relationship

I believe in the work relationship that whatever you do, do it to the best of your knowledge. Be respectful to people above and under you where you work. I believe that you have to be fair, impartial, and unprejudiced. Always work hard without discrimination and go above and beyond your call of duty or responsibility. Don't set a limit to time and assignment. Try very hard not to cave under pressure. Be calm and confident. Just take a deep breath and relax for a few second. Be confident and don't ever panic. Know that in every place you work, there is a test and trial time to assess your personality. Be honest, loyal, accurate, prompt, and not afraid of hard work. Remember to be yourself and not what others want you to be. And if you can't remain yourself and feel that you have to wear a different hat for different people because of a job, it's time to leave that job and look for another. Your health and your life are worth more than anything else. When it comes to integrity, I'd rather change a lot of jobs instead of compromising my right to be who I am. No! I am not going to change myself to please others with less morals and ethic sometimes. I know that promotion, raise, bonus, and early retirement or pension seems nice and tempting. But if I have to make the sacrifice of being someone that I am not, then nothing is worth it.

LOVE PARTNERSHIP AND RELATIONSHIP

Love Relationship

I believe that with some work, patience, kindness, and understanding, almost any relationship can work real well. The essential is to establish a good system of communication so that people can be on the same plan. That means not one person is in the North Pole and the other is in the South Pole.

I believe that any relationship needs mutual efforts, abilities, consensus, respect, consideration, and generosity in order to work and last a long time being happy together. I believe that both partners should be open-minded, free-spirited, forgiving, not holding grudge for each other if something does not work their way. They should not be controlling, demanding changes, not giving ultimatums, not dictating to each other, not taking over each other and not taking away from each other. They should not monopolize each other. Instead, they should complement each other.

People in a love relationship should be accepting of each other the way each one comes in the relationship without expectations of any kind. Therefore, there wouldn't be any surprise good or bad. If good surprises come, be glad, appreciate them and be grateful for them, pay a compliment, give a hug or a kiss to reward the person. Make sure that if the person asks "What for?" tell him or her right away what that was for. This will be a way to reinforce good behavior. If bad surprises come, accept them and work on solving the problems that cause them as a team.

I also believe that couples or people in a relationship should have common interests, should do a lot of activities together, and should be with each other as much as possible. I also believe that in a romantic relationship, either marriage or boyfriend or girlfriend, both partners should have these qualities in order to make it work real well and last for a long time. They should have a good sense of humor, know how to laugh, know how to have fun, be strong, and have good understanding. Above all, I believe that both partners should be frank, open, free to be themselves, be able to be an individual, able to do things with each other, for each other, or for himself and for herself. Also at times, they should be able to be on their own, be independent, assertive, initiate, and take good care of himself or herself. I believe that some decisions should be discussed. Nevertheless, if sometimes a partner takes the chance of being independent instead of interdependent and decide to do something, it should be fine too because a relationship is a partnership where people are equal. In any relationship, autonomy is needed. Partners have to provide autonomy, trust, and spontaneity instead of elaborating and calculating plans at all time.

I believe that in any relationship, people have to be in it completely in order to experience and to enjoy the fun and the beauty of it. For this to happen, partners need to be committed to each other. I believe that if people are afraid, have one foot in and the other out when going into a relationship, thinking how and when they are going to get out, they should not even be in at all. Because almost everybody can recognize nonverbal behaviors, they will not let each other in to prevent disaster. Just know that if one person is hiding something, not being completely honest and loyal, it will come out whether he or she wants it or not when it's least expected.

Business Partnership

I believe that in a business partnership, like in any other relationship, people should be open, honest, work hard, share ideas, discuss decisions before making them, communicate freely, and have long and short meetings often as needed. They should be respectful to each other and agree or disagree with each other. I believe that they should come to an agreement that is suitable and beneficial to the business as soon as possible. They should know that the business comes first and their private life and their problems should be completely out during meetings, at the workplace, and during work time.

I believe that in a relationship or business partnership, no other feelings should be involved. I believe that people definitely should not mix business with pleasure. When people are at work, they should work. And when they want pleasure or other feelings, they should go somewhere else with someone else who doesn't take part in the business partnership. The only partnership that can be related to other feelings or relationship is the one with family members, for example, husband and wife, father and son, mother and daughter, etc. To me, if the business place is different from the living place, other feelings should not be put on display in there.

Money: A Touchy Subject

I believe that money can cause a lot of problems in a relationship, especially when there is lack of it. Money can cause a lot of stress, which can turn to unhealthy situations. I believe that money comes with work, effort, action, sacrifice, and risk for spending it or having it first before you can make it. Even if you win the lotto, you have to have the $1, dress up, go to the store to buy the winning ticket, save it, then read it and know what to do with all the money that you had never handled before. You need to protect the money, yourself, your family, and know how to be happy with all this money. Otherwise, you can make some regrettable mistakes that can destroy you, your loved ones, and others if you don't know how to deal with the new situation.

I believe that if you were born into money it is different than newly acquired money. I believe it's important to have money to buy nice things for yourself and your loved ones because it's your money that you work hard for or your heritage to enjoy while you are alive and well or not. But I also believe that money shouldn't be spent crazily and needlessly. People should buy their needs such as health care, foods, shelter, clothing, and transportation and save some for rainy days and your loved ones' education, future, and in helping others who don't have any. I also believe that good, honest, loyal, and compassionate people are even more important to me than others with a lot of money because people with these qualities are so rare it seems they are almost impossible to find or are nonexistent. These qualities and the very few who possess them are priceless. Therefore, no money in the world can buy them.

The Government

I believe that rich people with a lot of money should help the poor people too instead of relying on the government solely to help them in all capacities. I believe there are some needs that become so imperative that we can't wait but help these people in our own little way. If we are not rich to do so in a big noticeable manner, we can do it per our possibility.

I believe that the government is an institution that people need in order to control chaos; set limits; enforce laws, rules, and regulation; and to protect the good guys from the bad guys and the bad guys from themselves. I believe that the government should be partial, fair, have concern for their citizens' welfare. I believe that like it or not, people should respect the laws, rules, and regulation enforced by the government. I believe that people should sometimes do what they can to help the government instead of expecting for the government to do all at all times for them. I also believe that people shouldn't criticize negatively what happens in the government sometimes. Instead, they should find out about a suggestion box or available online ways to convey their good ideas and suggestions, advices, and encouragement as needed to the government. Remember, we are the people; we are the ones making the government. Therefore, we are the government.

Three Social Groups

After my observation of people in society, I believe that there are figuratively three types or groups of people, which are the takers, the keepers, and the givers that I want to talk about in detail.

THE TAKERS

The takers take and take and take whatever they can from wherever they can see and find anything they can. They take from whoever they can without discrimination. They never pass opportunity to take whatever it is regardless of how they get it and who gets hurt from what they take. For the takers, everything is irrelevant except taking.

The takers take and take and take every year, every month, every week, every day, every hour, every minute, and every second. The takers take and take and take and never take enough no matter what title the takers have, how many billions of dollars the takers have, they are still taking from others who have close to none or very little to survive.

For your information, the takers take emotions, love, admiration, compassion, dignity, loyalty, integrity, kindness, attention, innocence, humility, pride. The takers take mentally also: knowledge, time, advice, intelligence, others' techniques, others' manners, creativity, talents, gifts, arts, others' hard work and pass them as their own.

The takers are like a fox. They can lure you, trap you, cry with you, laugh with you until you don't have any more for them to take. So they drop you on your face like an empty sack of potato and move on to other pastures. The takers take and take and never take enough to finally stop taking. If something, someone, or some circumstance did not stop them on time, they would have taken your heart and soul.

Therefore, people, open your eyes, ears and be aware of takers. People, stay away from takers if you don't want to be their victims. Sometimes in order to trick you, the takers pretend to be a giver. They give you compliments, flattery, cheap things that they get for free, fun, and temporary joy in order to obtain more from you than what they give to you. Just know that there are more takers than keepers and givers combined in our society. You don't even need an example at all to know the takers who are all around you night and day in any walks of life. Just pay attention and you will notice them. Because they are the majority and are living with you, near you, and around you. Whether you want it or not, if you are not careful, they can and will take from you.

THE KEEPERS

The keepers keep and keep and keep whatever they earn, whatever is given to them, or whatever was thrown away. The keepers use old clothes, shoes, bags, dilapidated furniture and keep every cent they make from work. The keepers usually work two jobs near home. Most of the time, the keepers make smart investments in real estate, which they can obtain easily. They usually have large amounts of cash on hand. And almost always they find beautiful homes on sale, auctions, and/or repossessed very cheaply. The keepers don't usually use loans or share with other people. Most keepers don't go anywhere, don't entertain, and don't have close friends or relatives around them. They work two jobs. Therefore, no one ever knows enough about them to get into their business. Often, the keepers look decrepit, unkempt, dressed with hand-me-downs and appear poor enough for you to feel sorry for them. Sometimes some look pretty decent, clean, and appropriately dressed in uniform or street clothes depending on what profession they are in or what kind of job they do. The way the keepers look sometimes can be very deceitful. Because most of the time the keepers are millionaires. And you wouldn't even know it if they don't tell you. Even when they tell you, you couldn't believe it unless they show you proof. The keepers keep and keep and keep everything and anything. So they don't have to spend a cent and keep all the money they make by working. Most keepers don't own a car, don't drive, don't go to the restaurant, don't go to entertainment places, and don't go to clothing stores or any store at all. The keepers work in places where they can get "freebies" to keep and use.

The keepers are usually friendly, respectful, polite, nice, and sweet people. Right now, you may know or see some keepers almost every day in your life because the keepers walk to and from work and many places they have to go. But if the keepers don't volunteer to tell you who they are and how much they are worth in dollars and cents or real state, you would never know.

My husband and I know many keepers who for some reason trust us to tell us about their wealth or riches. The keepers are very good employees; they keep their multiple jobs to make money to buy and keep homes. Some keepers are users too. They use whatever they can get for free to keep their money. It's not easy to explain the keepers. After the two examples of male and female keepers/users, you will be able to understand very well what I mean by keepers.

EXAMPLE A

Years ago, my family and I lived in Queens where we met a man named Rigal who walked in the neighborhood just like my husband and I. My husband and I said hello, and he said hello back to us. As time passed by, we knew a little more about him. We found out that he lived a few blocks away from us and worked two full-time jobs. One job was for the appliance industry. The other was living in as a super in a building of multiple apartments rented to rich people with good career-oriented professionals in well-paid jobs. This job came with a furnished four-bedroom apartment, paid utilities, appliances and garage included. Both jobs were well paid also.

Since he did a great job, was a polite, respectful, and a friendly person, all the tenants loved him and gave him almost everything he needed for himself, his wife, and his children (three boys). They gave him clothes when they changed their wardrobe, linens, kitchen utensils, dishes, furniture when the tenants remodeled their apartment, and holiday gifts of money, foods, appliances, gadgets, cosmetics enough for him and his family that he never had to spend a cent from his paychecks.

All this keeper had to say was thank you and be grateful, used, and kept everything given to them, piled his money in the bank, and bought two beautiful homes in Boston, Massachusetts, and four others in Queens, New York.

One day, my husband was driving home from work and saw him walking in the street from a good distance of two to three miles from home and offered him a ride. While riding in my husband's car, this keeper told him that he had more than one million dollars in the bank. My husband said, "No, you are kidding me. Are you joking!" He said, "No, man, I am not joking. I just came from the bank to make a deposit. See for yourself." My husband looked at the bankbook and noticed 1.5 million dollars with the date next to the deposit and his name on top of the page. My husband said, "How, did you win the lotto?" Mr. Rigal the keeper answered, "No, I just made the money from my salaries working in two well-paid jobs and no need to buy anything. One of the jobs as a super gave me free apartment, appliances, furniture, free utility, free car garage, which I rented because I had no car, free food, clothes, shoes, handbags for my wife, school supplies for my children, toys, gifts, money, and anything I needed, I got it from the tenants. Therefore, I had nothing to do with my salaries. All I have been doing is depositing some money in the bank. I bought six new beautiful homes with multiple apartments with cash and rented them out to rich people who took good care of them and mailed me my rent money on time every month.

"Since these homes are brand new, they don't need maintenance. And if they did, I could have done it myself as a handyman without spending a cent."

He further explained to my husband that his children went to public school two blocks from home. The tenants where he lived gave them clothes, shoes, schoolbags, supplies, toys, and games. "These tenants gave my wife all she needed also. We never had to buy anything we needed."

The catch is, this man never got sick and never used his two insurances to have a family doctor and annual checkups. One day in his late thirties, he had abdominal pain and went to a city hospital in the neighborhood, which was at walking distance. No questions were asked at the hospital except for his name, address, and what was wrong; and a staff member placed him on a stretcher and rolled him to a room for a doctor to see him. He was seen by a doctor who told him that he had a hernia and needed to be operated on by the end of the week. At the hospital, he received a painkiller and was told to go home and make arrangements to come back for surgery.

According to his appearance, the hospital staff treated him as an indigent. The staff never asked him for an insurance card, never charged him for anything. They just assumed that he was very poor and couldn't pay for anything. But the hospital personnel assigned medical students to operate on him as practice for their exams. These students made several costly mistakes during a simple hernia surgery. As a result, this keeper lost his life and kept all his money and wealth.

By that time, his three boys had become adolescents dropped out of high school, got into trouble, worked some time in menial jobs to provide for themselves, and lived in dilapidated homes in a poor neighborhood. After the father died, these children had the best surprise of their lives when a lawyer told them how many houses and how much money he had left for them.

My husband said to me, "Honey, if that was me in this keeper's place, I would ask to see the best surgeon and the best private hospital in the state of New York where students don't have to practice on me." "I would have made a deal with the doctor to pay him one-half of my one and a half million dollars and save my life and forget about the two medical insurances unused for twenty-five years." Not only did this keeper work two full-time jobs, his wife worked too, his children worked and made their own living at an early age without the parents. And remember the six beautiful multiple dwellings, only one could have saved his life by paying for the hospital, the surgeon, and private duty nurses as needed. Again, according to this keeper's appearance, everybody including his wife and children assumed that they were poor.

EXAMPLE B

A female keeper who worked with me in one of her two full-time jobs confessed her million dollars to me while passing as the poorest but sweetest employee of a medical facility. Not too long ago, I worked in a medical facility with a lady who got two full-time jobs, one in the medical field and the other in the educational field. At that time, she was a friendly, respectful, polite, helpful, peaceful, confident, and talkative person. She dressed clean and simple with a uniform and white jacket or lab coat. She drove a cheap old Japanese car and lived a few blocks from work. To go to the other job and back home, she rode the school bus. She ate all her meals from either job. At the school, she ate school food with the children. At the medical facility, she ate in the cafeteria from food for employees and leftover dirty trays after the patients finished their meals. One day, I tried to stop her but without success. I told her that the food tray that she picked up was a dirty one from a patient who had MRSA, a very contagious infection. But she answered, "I know, Marie, but I like chocolate cake and there was a piece on the tray that they left untouched." The following day, I worked with her, used the same phones, and sat close to her. She was covered with glue and slippery mucus from her nose and mouth. She sneezed and pulled phlegm for the entire evening. I gave her a few cups of my ginger and cinnamon tea with lemon juice that I had brought from home. She took two Tylenol tablets, adding them to the tea. When I got home that night, I drank some of my tea, gargled warm saltwater, ran a hot bath with alcohol in it, breathed the steam and threw all the clothes I wore in the washing machine with hot water, double rinsed and bleached them. I dried them for sixty minutes in hot heat. I threw away my shoes.

While working with this keeper/user, she told me that she was living in a kitchenette with her husband, didn't cook, didn't watch TV, didn't buy the newspaper, didn't go to entertainment, didn't buy foods, didn't own a computer, didn't have a telephone at home nor a cell phone. She told me that she brought foods home from work for herself and her husband. She used the computer at work to search the Internet. She watched TV at work, read the newspaper at work when someone left them, and made all her phone calls at work. If she got sick, she used medications at work and didn't even have to pay copayment from her two insurances of the two full-time jobs. She didn't have to buy almost anything except clothing, shoes, cosmetics, and pay rent that differentiated her from the male keeper in the previous example.

This person I worked with, this keeper/user, deserved the extra title "user" because besides keeping, she also used what was not hers. She told me, "Marie, I just bought a corner modern condo in a rich neighborhood for $800,000 cash from money I saved from my two jobs where I got almost everything for free." I said to her that she still have to pay for tax and maintenance. She answered, "I know, Marie, but I still have a lot of money in the bank for that." That was the last time I saw her. She was lucky that I was there to give her my tea from home. I hope she got luckier than the male keeper and keep her life instead of the money in the bank and the luxurious home.

THE GIVERS

Let us save the best for last. Out of the three types described in this chapter, the smallest one, which is the most wonderful, is the genuine giver. The givers give and give and give. The givers give love, affection, joy, smile, laughter, happiness, jokes, humor, fun, hugs, kisses, courtesy, attention, care, advices, compassion, compliments, time, ideas, confidence, self-esteem, encouragement, dreams, creativity, hope, desire, ambition, will, beliefs, positive attitude and criticism, good judgment, wisdom, counseling, solutions to problems, good thinking, the deepest sympathy, and empathy. When needed, some givers cry and mourn with you and even carry the burden for you.

Physically, the givers give material things too according to the needs. The givers give clothes, shoes, handbags, furniture, appliances, linen, foods, money, homes, cars, and almost everything possible for them to give to people in order to help. Materially and financially, some givers give and give and give until they only leave very little for themselves to survive. The best givers most of the time give others who turn out to have more and better than them. At that point, these givers feel the happiest and are the most fulfilled, peaceful, and grateful for what they have left for themselves. Sometimes the givers give their lives to save others who can be perfect strangers or loved ones.

In rare occasions or cases, the givers are misunderstood in giving love, affection, protection, safety net or blanket, good advices, and guidance that the receiver perceives as intruding to his or her privacy, disrespect, putting stress and bruising his or her ego or pride. Then the givers give the people who need their help a break duly until they fully comprehend their needs and situations that the givers wanted to ameliorate for them. It seems to me that most givers have intuition and a sixth sense to know exactly what to give to someone in immediate need.

Example C

I was walking in a mall near my house after dinner as usual. But I wasn't my normal self. I was thinking about how to solve some financial problems. I was down, dejected, and probably looked tired too. But I refused to pass my daily two hours of walking exercise. While walking, I noticed a new walker, a young lady who looked like twenty-five to thirty years old. I started to look at her from the bottom up because she was so tall with big bones and fit that I couldn't see her very well as a whole. She wore casual slacks, short-sleeved printed blouse, a sweater tied at the waist, and street-walking shoes. After I observed all the way past her waist, I decided to look at her face. That was a good decision. Because I noticed on her face the most spectacular, wonderful, beautiful, joyful, generous, given smile that I had never seen before in my life. She smiled with her eyes, her nose, her cheeks, her full lips, her white well-aligned glittering teeth, and her positive, generous, forward attitude that was targeted at me and for me that I couldn't resist or dare not to smile back at her.

That young lady's smile lifted me, brought me joy, encouragement, creativity, gratitude for what I have, perseverance on what I dream, solutions to my problems, emotional health, self-confidence, and a boost of energy that I really needed. After my walk, I went home and spent the entire evening cleaning my house, organizing my paperwork, my budget, and prioritized my bills. The next day, I went on the computer to continue writing this book that I stopped for a while. Up to now, whenever I think about this *young lady's smile at me and for me, I say to myself, "No, I can't go down and feel sorry for myself. I have to go up and stay up for the rest of my life."*

EXAMPLE D

I have one of my two sons asking me one day if I was okay and what happened. After answering yes I was okay, he left it just like that and went to his room. He stayed for a while there doing something that gave him a mischievous look on his face while coming back to me. I was sitting on the sofa in my living room working on my budget. I stopped and looked at him standing about three feet in front of me. As soon as I looked at him, he started acting up, twisting his body—hands, fingers, arms, shoulders, neck, face, lips, waist, back, legs, and feet—turning to an unknown earth character. He had a shrill made-up voice, and he talked his own language like a robot. I could not resist throwing away my budget book and my pen and bending over forward and backward, throwing my hands and legs up in the air simultaneously with a laughter that sounded like a thunder blast. Then I stopped laughing and calmed down. When I least expected it, my son started his own laugh. He started laughing all the way down from his belly, moved it up to his chest and throat like a shrill of aaaaaaaaaaAHAH while bending and stretching with all kinds of joyful expressions until the laugh rolled out of his mouth like a dynamite blast. I had never seen anything like that before in my life.

To compensate him for the wonderful gift, I told him to get a shower and dress casually. He did, and I did the same. When he was ready, I said, "Let's go to the amusement park, the Six Flags in New Jersey." We spent the entire evening riding, watching shows, participating in events, walking, eating, taking pictures, buying souvenirs, hugging and laughing together. We had the most wonderful time that we deserved.

Some of my children are givers and give different gifts. My husband and I are givers also. My husband and I give money, foods, education, tuition, a place to live for college students, family, and friends. I am afraid sometimes that if we are not careful enough, we might give too much and don't leave enough for us to survive. But we also give what money can't buy—we give care, attention, advice, counseling, time, help, assistance in construction work, appreciation, compliments, joy, and laughter for free to anyone who needs us.

About the types of people, this was my own philosophy coming from anyone or anywhere that I know. I made the categories up according to my observation. The examples are true. You don't have to agree with me if you don't want to. But feel free to have your own philosophy, your own made-up and observed group, which I would be glad for if you want to share it with me after you read this book; at the end of the book is where my phone number usually is.

All Sorts of Needs and Some Examples

Need for Affection and Empathy

There are many ways that you can show affection and empathy to people in such a need. It doesn't have to be on a big scale, with a large organization during the time of catastrophe or disaster. Sometimes you don't need lots of money and TV ads, or you might not even know why, how, or when and where to do it. Just do what your heart and soul tell you to do for others in need. Most of the time, it is not what the person wants or what you want. It is what the needs are.

Just be open-minded, alert, observant, honest, giving, and you will find out people's needs and how to help them. I have so many examples of needs that I provide to people without putting one cent out nor too much of my time either. There are also some examples that I can't even explain. These are some of the examples that I can explain:

Example Number 1

Need for Empathy and Compassion

As a child—I can't even remember exactly how old I was, probably eight or nine years old—I did something for someone who really needed it. I gave attention and empathy to a child who was around my age. There was a little girl approximately my age or even younger who used to shop in my parents' grocery store. She used to buy oil, rice, beans, and charcoal. In that store, we had produce from our farms mostly. But this little girl never shopped for them or anything else except for the items above.

By this girl's look, I could tell that she was poor, was from the countryside, not living with her parents, not having friends, not allowed to play and not being properly or adequately cared for. At that age, she already was working for a living. I noticed what time she shopped every day and made sure that I was in the store. When I was in the store, I gave her what she shopped for free of charge and gave her back the money. With the money and without a word, she picked up a piece of cake and some cookies. And with a big smile, she thanked me and left without a sound or word. She did it so I wouldn't get in trouble. Later on, I let her get the foods, the charcoal, the cake, the cookies, and the money too. I also followed her and saw where she lived with a divorced lady and two children, a boy and a girl older than her.

These older children went to school, the mother went to work in a factory, and there was no father or man there. The apartment was one large room divided by a moveable wooden divider with two beds into that space. One bed was for the mother and daughter, and the other for the son. I asked the little girl where she slept, and she answered here, pointing her finger at a spot on the other side of the divider. The running water and the kitchen were in a small porch in front of the house.

On the same porch, on one side was a sink made in cement. On the other side was a cooking area like a square made of bricks around an empty inside, which was like a barbecue pit. Inside it, the little girl placed the charcoal, lighted it by using pieces of paper that were very hard to light up because of the wind; but when it finally lighted up, it burned fast and bright red due to the oxygen outside. The little girl placed a deep black pot with a long handle on top like a pail with some water in it, washed some beans, and placed them in the pot to boil. While boiling, we talked and played with make-believe roles with mongo seeds.

That was our secret! If my mother knew, she would have stopped me from going to a place like that and being a friend to someone like her. My mother would have called social services, have this woman arrested for using a young child like that as a housekeeper and cook instead of sending her to school like her own children. On the other hand, if the lady or her children knew, the little girl would have been in trouble and be punished for letting a stranger in their secret life.

To that poor little girl, something terrible happened. One day, the little girl came to shop and I wasn't at the store. I stayed late to practice a school play.

She shopped for what she needed as usual, took the cake and the cookies, and didn't pay for the foods. The cashier took the foods back for nonpayment. Unfortunately, the cashier let her get the charcoal too. She went home, didn't finish her cake and cookies, was crying until the mother came back from work and the children from school were real hungry and screaming at her. There was no food to cook.

Next, the lady or mother made the little girl light a fire with the charcoal, pulled off her panties, and sat her down on top of the fire and placed a hand on her mouth. By the time the neighbors smelled the burning flesh and came out to investigate, it was too late for the little girl whose lower torso was burned, and she died before the ambulance and the police arrived. The lady got arrested, and the girl was sent to a juvenile delinquent facility. The boy was sent to foster parents.

I never forgot that little girl whom I never knew the name. Maybe she never knew my name too. We were so cautious of not letting others in on the secret that we used more actions than words. We communicated by our laughter, joy, play, and togetherness. We helped each other fulfill our needs so well that words weren't that important for us.

I was heartsick for a long time until I confessed to my mother what was wrong with me. And she supported me and never blamed me. My mother said to me, "Remember the joy, the laughter, the fun, the short period of happiness you gave and shared with that little girl when she was in need, and forget about what you couldn't do for her." Since then, I knew that needs could be many things and many ways, which are not necessarily material possessions.

Example Number 2

Need of Empathy and Trust

One day, I was in Northern Boulevard, Queens, New York, going somewhere. A few blocks from my house, I met a young lady embracing a pole and crying. I pulled her hands out of the pole, gave her a hug, and told her to come with me. I placed my arms around her to prevent her from falling until we got home. I sat her down, washed her face, and placed a cold compress on top of her puffy face, neck, and shoulders. I gave her some soup, juice, and water and two Tylenols after asking her if she was allergic to the drug and she said no. She ate and drank and stopped crying. When my husband got home from work, I placed my index finger to my lips while looking at him. Without a word, he understood and walked away from the living room where we were. When night came, I gave the lady clean towels, sheets, a blanket, a new nightgown. I showed her where the bathroom and the guest room were. On top of the bedside table, I placed two more Tylenols for her to take in the next few hours and a glass of water if needed.

For many days, I left her in the house with food already cooked, water, juice, milk, my work phone number, and money for a cab. I also told her that she didn't have to talk unless she was ready and really wanted to. I also told her not to go out. And if she had to go out, she should not intend to come back. I was afraid that the person who did this to her might follow her to my house.

After a few days, when the swelling went down, she told me that she had called some family members and let them know that she was alive and well. She told them that it was better for them not to know where she was. She knew that her husband was going to harass them to find out where she was. When she was ready to leave my house, she asked me to help her find a job and rent a place to live in a different city. I did find her a job, found her a one-bedroom apartment, and provided her the money for rent, furniture, clothes, and shoes until she got on her feet.

After a few months, she came to visit me unannounced. When I opened the door, I didn't recognize her. She told me when I asked that she was the lady I helped a few months ago. She looked so nice. She gave me a beautiful embroidered tablecloth that she made for me. She told me that she was from a West Indian island called Dominica, a member of the West Indies Associated States. She spoke Patois and Creole from the French who occupied her country long ago. She told me that the day I saved her, she was beaten by her jealous husband. She said, "I had a childhood male friend that happened to be in the United States, who got my address from relatives and paid me a surprise visit." Her husband got home early, found the visitor, didn't ask questions, grabbed him by the throat, and threw him out in the street. He turned to her and beat her to a pulp with his fists. He left her for dead. She passed out for some time, came through, scrambled outside, and hugged the electrical pole where I found her that particular day six months ago. She said thank you and wanted to pay me. I said, "You don't have to, it wasn't a loan. You are welcome, good luck, and take care of yourself." I never knew her name, didn't bother to ask. I don't think she knew mine either. I didn't know her address (she got the place from a real state) and didn't know her phone number either. I didn't intend to communicate with her so she wouldn't feel obligated to me.

Example Number 3

Need for a Hug and Reassurance

In 2005, I was supervising in a Long Island nursing home when the ambulance brought a homeless man that I noticed while making rounds. The nursing staff was already prepared for the admission. I stopped in the room anyway ahead of the team members. When I saw this dirty and smelly man, I was caught by his unusual facial expression, which was pure fear. The man was petrified and very scared. His entire body cramped and recoiled. And his eyes were wide open. Right away I dismissed the team, closed the door, and turned off the bright light. I bent over this scared man, placed both hands around him, picked him up, and hugged him. I told him in a soothing voice, "Don't be afraid. We are here for you, we are on your side, and we love you and will take good care of you. All you have to do is relax and let us help you." I turned on the bright light, took his vital signs, undressed him, dressed him with a clean gown, gave him a glass of water, and looked at the paperwork. I found out that this man I was hugging closely to my bosom had meningitis, a very contagious disease. But it was too late for me anyway who was cleaning and bending over him, wiping his runny nose and breathing his breath without precautions. I didn't get sick, but I had an open, relaxed face and a faint smile from him.

What this man really needed was reassurance, to feel secured, have emotional comfort and compassion more than anything else at that time to be in his way to recovery. By the time we (the team) called the doctors to get medication orders for him and got his medications from the pharmacy, the supplies to install his IV antibiotic, he was already relaxed, clean, smelled good, and looked better than when he came. Next we ordered food from dietary and had a social worker and recreational therapy and whatever he *needed to make a pleasant stay and complete recovery before leaving the place. The fear, the bad smell, the dirty clothes, the runny nose, the thirst, and the hunger were all gone in less than an hour. They were all replaced by confidence, smiles, and peace because of the initial act of a simple hug, reassurance, and security that was needed by this very scared man.*

These needs are smaller but very important because they are physical:

Need for Medical Care

To let a person who is sick and in pain be chased out of a hospital because this person's insurance had run out or he doesn't have one at all is denying the gift of life to this individual.

Example Number 4

In 2009, in a Brooklyn, New York, county hospital, a poor woman didn't have a friend or relative to accompany her to the emergency room while she felt sick. She got herself together and went to the emergency room, but she didn't have enough energy to find an employee to direct her to where she needed to go and find the forms to fill out. She sat in the large emergency room for thirty-six hours without food, medical care, and water and in pain. She passed out, fell to the floor until the cleaning person found her and reported to the personnel. "Come fast, there is a lady on the floor." She was unnoticed in a crowded city emergency room until she died.

I know firsthand what being in pain means because sometimes I choose to stay with the pain although I could have taken a painkiller or run to the emergency room for help. But I didn't take the painkiller or run to the emergency room to get help from the doctors. I didn't do all of the above not because I didn't have health insurance, the money to pay copayment, or someone to accompany me to the emergency room. The reason is I was tired of it and because it wasn't effective and I wanted to see how long I could hold on without a painkiller. I want to find out what can I do to stop the pain, what caused it in the first place, and why that pain couldn't be diagnosed. This pain that I refer to is in my previous book named T.H.A.T.S., The Health Assistance to Some. *I had abdominal pain between digestion and elimination due to bacteria in my unprotected food before I knew in depth* about the food protection program of the health department. This was what inspired me to make my own health program T.H.A.T.S.

Need for Foods to Eat and Water to Drink

Eating and drinking are vital for people who don't have food and water. For people who have these two, it's nothing. Some people have so much foods that they can never finish eating them and have to throw away some of them while others can't find enough or any at all for the entire day and not be able to sleep at night because they are too hungry. Why don't some people make it their business to share their foods with people who don't have instead of relying solely on the government to do so? People can help through a charity, some organizations, but it would be faster and more direct in if it was in their own neighborhood. Just by paying attention and observing what is going on next door, you can see little children coming from school locked out until other family members get home to open for them. If you witness something like that, call the child, let him or her sit inside your house and offer some snacks until someone arrives. Take the child yourself and explain what you did voluntarily so the child wouldn't get in trouble with other family members.

Sometimes both parents in a family need to work two jobs to pay the mortgage, utility bills, heating for the home, and buy foods, clothing, etc., for their children. When you see something like that, ask what you can do to help. Or offer a tray of hot, healthy foods ready and cooked enough for the family. They might accept it or not. So what if they are too proud to accept your help? It cost you nothing. You can always divide the foods in many small portions and store it for your own family. Or they might accept it, enjoy it, and be grateful to you. No matter what way it went, this act didn't take from you. It added to you for doing a good deed. My husband and I know real well what it means to be hungry even though it's by choice. We are both workaholics. So when we start a project, we want to stop only when we complete it.

Most of the time, the project takes a long time and we get hungry. By the time we get to the kitchen, open the refrigerator and the microwave at the same time, we become ravenous and bump into each other. After one of us made concession and said, "You first" and stopped all activity, then we could *function. He or she let the other person fix his or her food and sat down by the table to eat. The other person did the same activity of food fixing and sat down by the same table also. After we both finish eating and drinking, my husband said to me, "Honey, did you realize what just happened?" I said, "Yes! How hard and painful that is to be hungry." My husband said that although we have the food, we know where to find it and don't even have to cook it, just take it from the container, put it on a plate with a fork and a spoon, cut it with a knife, and place it in the microwave to heat up for a very short time; it makes us look so different. Now, can you imagine people that don't know where the food is coming from, don't have the food, don't see the food, probably going to spend the day and night without hope of eating some food at all. I answered, "I can and want to imagine, so I can see how blessed and fortunate we are, and I can make it my business to give food or a few dollars to someone who need food to eat." Besides organized charities, my husband and I go the old-fashioned way by sharing a plate of hot food or a bowl of hot soup we just made with a neighbor with young children regardless of what the neighbor might have. He or she might not have the time to order or prepare the food after work and like us need to eat or feed the children right away.*

Therefore, if you have more than enough ready-cooked food for yourself, offer the little more or extra to someone else. Don't wait for the food to go bad and throw it in the garbage. Share it with someone while it is good, fresh, and nutritious. Just tell the person, "This is good food I just made for myself, but I think it's a little too much for me alone. If you want, we can eat it together or we can share it. If you don't want it, don't be embarrassed to say no, I can keep it for the next day."

Sometimes my husband says, "Honey, why did you cook so much food for only the two of us? Take some food to the neighbors and I will take some to my coworkers. We can't waste so much good food." Other times, the neighbors my husband referred to happened to be new people who just moved to the neighborhood. Therefore, I replied, "I don't know if I want to share my foods with these people who are strangers to me. These people don't know us yet and might feel offended by our offer. May be after I present myself to them, I will try to share my foods with them." My husband agreed and took a big cooler full of ice and placed some good, healthy, and ready-cooked foods in it to bring to work and share with coworkers. My husband and I cook large amounts of good food that are high quality and fresh produced—poultry, fish, beef—all natural and organic, cage free, free range, free from growth hormones, pesticides, antibiotics, and chemicals. We used no stressed and tranquilized animals, no vegetables and fruits grown in fertilizer or sprayed with insecticide, pesticide, and covered with wax. We don't use artificial coloring, saturated fat, or trans fat. We only use vegetable oil and olive oil. We cook from scratch, even our desserts. The foods are also protected according to the food protection program from the U.S. Health Department.

What my husband and I care for is to prevent people from having hunger pains, eating contaminated foods from takeout places, or waiting for food delivery from a far place and eating spoiled foods from a vending machine. This is our way of providing a home-cooked meal for a family to eat together safely without taking away anything from us. It's very little for some people, and we wish that we could do it in a larger way. But it's better than nothing at all. At least, we acknowledge by our own experience the suffering that people can go through without food to eat even if it's temporary. We used food from our garden or from the farmers' garden where we can see the farm. Foods that we don't know too much about where they come from, like seafood and fish, we decrease our consumption of them.

Need and Example Number 5

Need for Shelter

This need is out of my league because I don't have enough money to do anything with helping people pay their mortgage. But I wish I could. When I see people being thrown out of their homes because of inflated adjustable mortgage that they can't pay, I feel heartsick. People need a place to live beside caves underground, tents, and sidewalks and shelters. People need at least an apartment with a kitchen to prepare their foods and for other commodities.

Need for Safety

People need safety in the streets and at home from robbers and killers. People can organize block association, patrol and community meetings, and private organization and security to protect them against racial and sexual discrimination, also from natural disaster, besides the government police.

Need for Education

Some higher education like city colleges or community colleges should be for free because the high school graduates' curriculum is not enough to get neither a good job nor knowledge to manage their lives, maintain relationships, and be able to communicate with people, budget their finance, and raise their children. Some people before graduation already owe so many loans they can't even stay until graduation. They are forced to quit but still have to repay the loan with high interest and nothing to show for it.

That was an idea of what I believe, my wisdom and philosophy about needs, and how people can help each other when in need without going out of their usual ways.

ABOUT T.H.A.T.S. PROGRAM

Before I start with the diseases and food and techniques to treat them, I would like to give the readers some recommendations about food protection and infection control by the United States Health Department. Please read the previous book named T.H.A.T.S., The Health Assistance to Some, *for great details to fully comprehend these two subjects.*

RECOMMENDATIONS

The following are some recommendations that I would like, you, the readers, to follow if you hadn't read the previous book T.H.A.T.S. *This reading can help you derive some good information that you need in order to fully understand and benefit from the reading you are doing now in* Food for Health and Cure. *Again, just know that there is a program with a book named* T.H.A.T.S. *In this program, I mentioned all foods that contain bacteria and other organisms, such as fungus, molds, viruses, parasites, worms that can be deactivated with ice, refrigerator, freezer, cold temperature storage before and shortly after cooking. We all need foods to survive, to be healthy, and to be energetic. Animal and their products contain the most dangerous and the most common bacteria. Some of them are more dangerous than the others. We need to eat animals and their products for our primary source of protein because most of us are not vegans or vegetarians. Even the vegetarians eat eggs, cheese, and drink milk. Only a very few of us are strictly vegetarians and find their protein in beans, soy, and nuts, which contain less bacteria. Therefore, when dealing with animals and their products, be very careful and follow these steps:*

1. *Buy your animals and their products in a place near home. Make sure that you pick them up from refrigerators or freezers.*
2. *Don't take too long to get home. Put them in refrigerators or freezers as soon as possible, meaning twenty minutes or less.*
3. *Place the frozen meat or animal products on the bottom shelf of the refrigerator the night before to defrost. Don't thaw these animal products on the table or the countertop.*
4. *Make sure that raw meat, poultry, and fish or other animal don't touch each other or other foods. The reason is cross contamination. Also, each one of the animals and their products has a different cooking time and a different cooking temperature that must be reached in order to be safely cooked. The animals and their products have a different storage temperature and process.*
5. *Wash working surfaces, utensils, cutting boards, and your hands before and after touching raw animals and their products. For touching meat poultry and fish, wear latex, plastic, or rubber gloves, if possible, to protect your hands from bacteria in the raw foods and to protect the foods from bacteria and viruses from your hands. Wear serving gloves in serving all foods to others.*
6. *Remember that your hands, washed or not, contain bacteria and viruses that you don't want to go into your food. And the foods contain bacteria that you don't want to go through your pores into your body via your hands. Food is only supposed to go to your digestive system.*
7. *To serve cooked food to other people, wear serving gloves or use napkins to touch all foods because you need a barrier between the food and you. The bacteria on your hands are incompatible with theirs. We all have our own bacteria in our body, which don't like other bacteria in someone else's body and can make someone else sick—even the people you love.*
8. *Cook all meat and animal products thoroughly by following instructions on the packages. Know how long to cook each type*

of food. And for more information about time to cook, read the T.H.A.T.S. *book.*

9. *Have a cold thermometer handy in your refrigerator at all times to control the cold temperature, which is between thirty-five to forty degrees Fahrenheit. Just read what is in it. You can buy it in hardware stores, supermarkets, and the kitchen section in department stores. Have a hot thermometer to check your cooked food for readiness and to deactivate bacteria from waking up and multiplying in your foods.*

10. *Keep hot foods hot and eat them hot. Keep cold foods cold and eat them cold.*

11. *Leftover foods should be discarded or stored in the refrigerator or freezer only if you know how to do that. Even in the refrigerator, leftovers should only be stored for twenty-four hours if they contain meat or animal products. Other foods can be stored and can last up to a maximum of three days at the most. If you want leftovers to be stored and used for more than twenty-four hours or three days, they will have to go in the freezer in small containers for one use at a time.*

12. *Do not store hot food in the refrigerator or the freezer. Let the food cool off for no more than twenty minutes. If the leftovers or the foods you want to store are still hot after fifteen minutes, you will know already that another five minutes is not going to cool it off. Therefore, you will have to speed up the process by placing the food on a large and flat tray and vent it with a paper plate or some napkins. Better yet, you can place cold, clean water, with ice cubes if needed, in another large container or tray and place the food in a smaller container or bowl, then put it on top of the tray with the cold water until it cools off.*

13. *Again, for your own safety, read the labels for safe handling instructions when you buy and prepare all foods, especially animals and their products. Look for approval seals or words like "inspected," "expiration date," "FDA," "USDA," and "inspected and passed" because all foods contain bacteria that can cause illness if the product is mishandled, stored, and cooked improperly. For your protection, when handling foods, follow the instructions that you acquired from* T.H.A.T.S. *food protection program in the previous book.*

14. *Know that chemicals in the foods slow down the bacteria but slow down your system also because you don't really have all the nutrients that you should if the food was naturally protected by physical protection.*

15. *We all need to eat a variety of foods for energy, health, and life. But don't forget that the same food without knowledge of preparing it properly can cause weakness, illness, and death. In this case, what you don't know can hurt you.*

16. *If you want to stay young, live long, be energetic, be healthy, be completely free from diseases, and be mentally, emotionally, and physically fit and happy, seek knowledge about foods from T.H.A.T.S. program. Just know that there is a food to cure, prevent, and/or ameliorate almost everything that you can have. You need to know which one to use for what you have or what you don't want to have. Prevention is better. Sometimes, we know from our genetic predisposition that we could have a disease that runs in the family. As soon as we find out, we should start to modify our diet to the foods that are beneficial to us in order to prevent this disease. And usually, it's not guaranteed that we are going to have that disease no matter what we do. If you are sick, your diet can help a great deal, in addition to medication and other medical procedures if you have no choice.*

17. *Some diseases can be controlled without medication or with less medication if you know what to eat and drink. You do not have to treat with medication everything you have. Sometimes you only have to eat certain foods, drink certain liquids, and follow certain techniques and activities.*

18. *Buy your food fresh from farms, supermarkets, or your own garden. Cook your food from scratch, and if you don't know how, this book will have some recipes. The previous book that you know already has some recipes, and you can buy a cookbook if you have to.*

19. *Stay away from foods cooked with preservatives or chemicals when you can only recognize three ingredients on the label that has twenty names that are not foods at all. If you see three names that you know as food, such as flour, eggs, and sugar on a cake's package and seventeen that you don't know, then stay away from that thing. Hungry or not, don't buy it.*

20. *Buy a cookbook and enjoy preparing your food. Use good judgment and your five senses. Eat moderately, be active, laugh a lot, follow*

what is in this book under what you have and what you don't want to have or just to stay healthy, live longer, or healthier with what you are about to learn from this book.

21. *Know that your health depends on what you eat, how you eat, how much you eat, and when you eat. Because the above is what keeps you alive and well or makes you sick and kills you. What you eat, how much you eat, and when you eat can prevent diseases or fight them. It can control your weight and keep you at your ideal weight, which in turn will cure or prevent a lot of diseases that will be covered in detail for each one in other chapters. Because obesity is responsible for many new diseases and conditions.*

22. *Just know that every single food you eat is either good or bad for something. That is why you need knowledge. And if you don't know about food, don't eat too much of anything so that you don't hurt yourself too much. Use moderation until you finish reading this book or the chapter that contains the disease you want to prevent, cure, ameliorate, or control with fewer medications.*

23. *Be alert and interested about foods. Investigate, pick up clues, practice your findings, experiment with foods, and have your own experiences with foods by not just cooking and eating them, but also by knowing about their goods and drawbacks. After reading these two books, watch programs referring to cooking. Criticize and collect information by reading other good books and magazines and going to seminars, lectures, and presentations, or meeting places where food is concerned and compare your knowledge of foods with others. Pat yourself on the back and be proud to observe how many mistakes some people make in preparing or cooking food now that you know about foods and their protection.*

24. *Remember, we are blessed to be in a beautiful and rich country like the United States, where some of us can find so many foods to eat that we have to be careful not to harm ourselves. Our government provides us with food protection or safety such as inspectors, USDA seals of approval, FDA daily allowances, food charts and pyramids, nutritionists, nutritional advice and guidance, and scientists and doctors to teach us about food. All you have to do is pay attention and learn. Everything is done for you, from the farms, the plants, all the way to the supermarkets or the stores where you buy the foods. Almost all foods are chemically or physically protected for you at this*

point. The rest is up to you to continue the same way on your way to your home, tables, and plates.

INFECTION CONTROL

The Health Department has infection control, the medical profession has infection control, and the food protection program has infection control for food. Infection control for food has become a part of the T.H.A.T.S. program, which is the only one that is discussed in this book.

Almost everyone has an idea about infection control and uses it in his own way. People usually wear gloves to wash dishes, cars, floors, pets, and hair and to clean the house and yard and pick up the garbage or trash. But they wash their foods with bare hands and prepare the foods with bare hands. They touch the cooked or raw food inside and outside of the pots and pans, serve them without serving gloves, and sometimes after touching money at the cash register. Other times, I observed people touching their nose, teeth, or private parts or scratching their scalp and pulling or twirling their hair and not washing their hands, not wearing gloves before touching other people's foods or their own.

For almost ten years, while building this program, I observed that most people, in person or on TV shows, rarely wash their hands or wear gloves before or after touching and serving food. Hands should be washed before and after touching foods, cooked or raw. People should wear gloves to prepare and serve foods. Hands should be washed before and after wearing gloves. Gloves are not an excuse for not washing hands. Gloves add a barrier. But when dealing with infection control, nothing can replace hand washing with liquid soap and warm water in sink or a washbasin for at least fifteen seconds. When dealing with foods, hands should be washed and dried before cooking and serving foods even if you wear gloves. Foods should never be touched by anyone with bare hands, especially for others. If you are cooking for yourself, maybe you can take the risk of using bare hands because you can get sick too by touching your own foods with dirty and ungloved hands from your own viruses, bacteria, mold, fungi, and worm eggs, which can go inside of you and hatch.

Some cooks or chefs, I have observed, usually taste the food with the same spoons that they put back in the pots full of cooked foods. They actually place the full spoon of food in their mouth with their saliva, tongue, and streptococci in their throat and return it to the rest of the food in the pot to mix with the food left in the pot for others to eat. I can't believe it that people are still doing these things in the year 2010.

People should know to take a small bowl or saucer, place the food to be tasted in it, get a spoon or fork, taste the food, and discard the rest. The tasting utensils and bowl or saucer should go in the sink to be washed and never again touch the rest of the food in the pot to be eaten by other people.

For more information about infection control of foods and diseases, please refer to the first book T.H.A.T.S., The Health Assistance to Some, *which is already published and you can purchase in the Web site Mariethats.com or at other Web sites and bookstores.*

LIST OF DISEASES/CONDITIONS

Abscess
Acidosis
Acne
Adrenal problems
Aging and prevention
Alcoholism
Allergy
Alzheimer's disease
Anemia
Anorexia
Anxiety
Arteriosclerosis
Arthritis
Asthma
Bedsores/decubitus
Bladder infection
Breast cancer
Breast-feeding problems/mastitis
Bronchitis
Bulimia
Burns

Bursitis
Cancers (some)
Canker sores
Cardiovascular disease
Celiac disease
Cirrhosis of the liver
Circulatory problems
Cold
Constipation
Cystic fibrosis
Dandruff
Depression
Dermatitis
Diabetes
Diarrhea
Drug addiction (substance abuse)
Dry skin
Edema
Embolism
Eye problems
Food-borne/water-borne illness
Fungal infection
Gall bladder disorders
Gout
Growth problems
Hair loss
Halitosis (bad breath)
Headache
Heartburn (gastro esophageal reflux)
High blood pressure (hypertension)
High cholesterol
Hepatitis (A, B, C)
Hyperthyroidism
Hypothyroidism
Hyperglycemia/hypoglycemia
Impotence
Immune system problems
Indigestion

Inflammation
Insomnia
Irritable bowel syndrome
Kidney disease
Kidney stones
Leg ulcer
Manic depressive disorder/ bipolar
Mood disorder
Memory problems
Menopausal and premenopausal problems
Migraine
Muscle cramps
Nail problems
Nasal congestion
Obesity
Osteoporosis
Peptic ulcer
Periodontal disease
Pneumonia
Prostate cancer
Smoking dependency
Skin disorders
Stress
Thrombophlebitis
Tuberculosis
Ulcerative colitis
Overweight and underweight or weight loss
Vaginitis
Warts
Worms (parasites)
Wrinkles

REMEDIES/THERAPIES

Enema
Exercise
Fasting
Light therapy

Music and sound therapy
Dance therapy
Belly dancing
Biofeedback
Breathing exercises
Guided imagery
Hypnotherapy
Massage
Meditation imagery
Relaxation techniques
Yoga, calisthenics exercises

ABSCESS

Abscess is a localized collection of pus in any part of the body, the result of disintegration or displacement of tissue. When pus accumulates in a tissue, organ, inside or outside of the body, an abscess is formed. An abscess may be the result from infection or inflammation. Most of the time, infections are the cause of the abscesses. Infections can be bacterial, viral, fungal, or parasitic.

A boil is an external skin abscess. For some abscesses, the area may become swollen, inflamed, hot, red, tender, itchy, and very painful. The person affected can experience fatigue, fever, chills, loss of appetite, and weight. Sometimes, blood infection and rupture of the abscess can happen. The materials inside of the abscess are usually from live and dead white blood cells, dead tissue, bacteria and their toxins, which need to be cleaned out of the body.

Acute Abscess

An acute abscess is an abscess with local symptoms of inflammation, with fluctuation and pointing about to rupture, also pressure and constitutional symptoms. Inflammation becomes intensified with increased heat, redness, swelling, and edema. Pain becomes throbbing and greater, with impaired loss of function of that part of the body. An elevation appears with fluctuation and softening; as it reaches the surface, it becomes necrotic and yellowish, giving way with evacuation of pus. Pressure symptoms are according to size and depth. Usually after the release of pus, the pain is decreased.

Abscesses in the floor of the mouth or neck, swelling may cause dyspnea and dysphagia. Constitutional symptoms vary from slight temperature, fever may be absent in a well walled-off abscess to high temperature with chills and sweats if associated with pyemia and septicemia. Any or general symptoms may be absent in deep-seated abscess except loss of weight and strength eventually.

The abscess may be terminated by pointing, evacuation and discharge of pus. Or it may become insipissated, encapsulated, and at times absorbed. The acute abscess appears suddenly and lasts a few hours, such as overnight, and gone the next day.

Chronic Abscess

Chronic abscess are the ones with pus but without signs of inflammation. They are usually of slow development. They are formed by liquefaction of tuberculosis tissue. They may occur anywhere on the body, but more frequently in the spine, hips, genitourinary tract, and lymph glands. Symptoms may be very mild. Pain when present is caused by pressure upon surrounding parts. Tenderness is often absent. Chronic septic intoxication with afternoon fever may occur. Amyloid disease may develop if the abscess persists for a prolonged period.

Chronic abscesses have been present for a long period of time such as days, weeks, even months. They are more resistant to treat because they cause more severe damage. When treated, the chronic abscesses begin to heal in a few days. Complete healing should happen between one to three weeks at the most unless there is a complication that can be bleeding or reopening of the abscess. But that does not happen frequently.

The names or types of abscess go according to where they are or what organs they appear at or on what part of the body they are formed. The following are some names of abscesses and where they are:

Alveolar Abscess

This is an abscess in the root of a tooth in the alveolar cavity, usually the result of necrosis and infection of dental pulp following dental caries. See your dentist right away. If you can't wait for appointment, do the following:

1. *Get a cup full of hot water and a half teaspoon of table salt. Drop it in the hot water and stir with the same spoon and let it cool off until you can comfortably hold a mouthful and gargle it vigorously for at least one minute. Repeat the process three times, which will give you three minutes per cupful. Stand by your washbasin and spit the contents after each gargle. Wait for two hours and repeat the same.*

2. *If after repeating the process for at least four times for the day and you still have pain, take a few whole cloves, chew them, or if not, smash them with the back of a spoon and place the paste on top of the abscessed area.*

3. *If you can't eat solid food yet, eat soup, mashed potato, mashed spinach, powdery low-fat cheese and low-fat milk, whole-grain spaghetti cut really small and drink homemade lemonade with fresh lemons and dark brown pure sugarcane.*

4. *By the time of your appointment, you will be fine already because this type of abscess don't last too long with this treatment.*

5. *To promote healing and preventing further occurrence, eat fresh fruits and vegetables of all colors: blueberries; strawberries; blackberries; apples; grapefruits; oranges; purple plums; red, black, and green grapes; tomatoes; and kiwis. As for vegetables, eat eggplants, leafy greens such as kale, collard greens, romaine lettuce, bell peppers of all colors, carrots, sweet potato, squash, onions, cabbage of all colors for vitamins and enzymes.*

6. *For protein, eat lean chicken, turkey, and lean beef, organic and natural; drink low-fat or fat-free milk; eat fat-free or reduced-fat cheese and yogurts with vitamin D, A, calcium, and other minerals.*

7. *Drink water, tea with ginger and cinnamon to decrease inflammation and infection. Vitamin C and protein can protect and repair damage tissue or cells and fight infection and diseases.*

True Story

In April of 2009, my husband and I went to the Pocono for vacation. During the second day of the seven days' vacation, my husband started to have pain by a molar (large back tooth). I offered a Tylenol tablet, which he refused. My husband told me that he could take the pain and didn't need any medication. But while shopping for food, the pain increased and an abscess developed.

In the same supermarket, we bought a box of salt and a jar of whole cloves. We made it home. At home right away, he heated up a cup of water in the microwave, added the half teaspoon of salt in it and shook it in his mouth and held it for a few minutes. Next, he mashed the cloves with a can of tomato sauce and placed the paste on the tooth and held it for another few minutes and took it off. After a few hours, he was able to call the dentist to make an appointment, which was a few days from the day he called because nothing was available before that date. Surprisingly, he spent the rest of the day without pain. And he slept well that night, woke up in the morning, practiced his workout exercises, ate breakfast, and forgot all about the pain.

The following day still, he had no pain and no discomfort. But he thought that he needed to continue the same treatment with the hot saltwater and the mashed cloves. While taking out of the cabinet the stuff needed for the treatment, he realized just on time that if he didn't have pain, why do the treatment? He stopped right there and enjoyed the rest of the vacation.

When we returned home on Sunday night, he slept well and still had no pain even after brushing and flossing the night before his appointment. On Monday morning, he went to the dentist and explained the pain and the abscess, thinking that he might need a root canal. Guess what? The dentist found no abscess, no cause for the pain, no infection, no cavity in that tooth, and no need for root canal because my husband had a root canal already from the same tooth.

Since that day, I made sure that he ate half of a large red or pink grapefruit daily, drank fresh homemade lemonade twice a week, adding to the very nutritious meals that we were eating already. I also increased his weight lifting in his daily workout that I made for him.

Amoebic Abscess of the Liver

This is an abscess occurring in the liver and developing as a complication of amoebic dysentery caused by Entamoeba histolytica.

Treatment

Eat fresh fruits, vegetables, whole-grain breads, cereals, pastas, lean meat, poultry, fish, tofu, and nuts and beans. Drink soybean milk, chocolate milk, tea, coffee sparingly and red wine too. Cut down on sodium and salt and concentrated sweets, and stay away from saturated animal fats and hydrogenated or trans fat from vegetable oil. Drink bottled water seven to eight eight-ounce cups per day. Use food protection and infection control from the other book T.H.A.T.S., The Health Assistance to Some *to prevent infection and contamination. Practice good hand washing with warm water and mild liquid soap in a sink or washbasin for at least fifteen minutes, many times a day as needed; use barriers between foods and bare hands and to touch everything dirty. Use sunscreen, clean your house, place soiled garments in a closed hamper, disinfect objects with alcohol, use sunlight and open window with screen to let oxygen in and purify the air exchanged.*

All the above can prevent you from having this disease, help you cure it if you already have it, and promote the healing process faster if you are recuperating.

ANORECTAL ABSCESS

This is an abscess in the tissue near the rectum; "ischiorectal" and "perirectal" are other names for this very painful, uncomfortable, and feeling ennui abscess. The area must be washed with clear warm water and mild liquid soap. Air should be provided periodically to allow oxygen interaction with this type of abscess, and light should be provided also because these types of abscess are caused by anaerobic bacteria that don't like light, oxygen, or air and open space. Bacteria in general, whether aerobic or anaerobic, like the dark, being free from air or oxygen and moist. Therefore, keep all abscesses dry and open to air or oxygen and plenty of light.

Next, apply lubricant, ointment, or cream provided by a doctor or OTC, over the counter, with the help of a pharmacist if no doctor has been consulted.

Nevertheless, with or without a physician, a good nutrition and activity can carry oxygen-rich red blood cells to every area in people's bodies, which can cure and prevent this condition regardless of what part of the body it is located.

Nutrition or Diet

Avoid fatty, processed, fried junk food; empty carbohydrate engineered foods; contaminated and infected food; chemical- and bacteria- and germ-laden foods.

Eat plant fat, no hydrogenated or partially hydrogenated oil, no saturated animal fat or oil. Use canola, olive, almond, flaxseed oil. Eat less animal products and more plant foods. Eat baked, boiled, grilled, and steamed food cooked by you. Eat organic and natural whole grains and fresh fruits, such as kiwi, apple, grapes, plum, nectarine, tangelo, oranges, grapefruits, melons, cantaloupe, bananas, pears, all the berries and pineapples. Eat green leafy vegetables, onions, celery, cabbages of all colors, bell peppers of all colors, carrots, squash, sweet potato, avocado, and nuts. Eat lean meat, poultry, fish and seafood, tofu, soy, and beans for fiber. And drink fresh lemonade, 100 percent fruit juices, fat-free milk, soy milk, chocolate milk, and yogurt. Drink eight eight-ounce cups of bottled spring water a day.

APICAL ABSCESS

This abscess at the apex of the lung is a very bad one because of the place it chooses. You can't reach there manually. But again with good nutrition, food that are protected from organisms, contamination, infection, full of nutrients, vitamins and minerals that can boost your immune system, you can fight, prevent, and cure this disorder. Sometimes you might need medical intervention or help. For food or nutrition details, follow the diet for previous conditions or abscesses.

APPENDICUALR ABSCESS/APPENDICIAL ABSCESSl

This abscess is due to the collection of pus or formation of it around an inflamed vermiform appendix. This abscess, of course, is inside of people and can't be seen or touched except through X-ray or surgery. But again, with high fiber from whole grain, fresh vegetables, such as cabbage, broccoli, kale, eggplants, and all leafy green vegetables and fresh fruits with fiber and vitamins and enzymes and minerals, you can fight this abscess or prevent it too. Remember, no fat, fast-food, junk, contaminated, infected foods should be eaten by anyone with this abscess. You should only consume fresh produce, lean dairy, lean protein from beef, poultry, fish, beans, nuts, avocado, olive oil, flaxseed, and canola oil, tea, omega-3 fatty acids and fish oil, and tomato sauce to prevent, cure, or ameliorate this condition after seeing your doctor or having surgery if needed.

ARTHRIFLUENT ABSCESS

Arthrifluent abscess is a wandering abscess having its origin in a diseased joint. If it is somewhere that you can see and touch, apply a cold compress made of ice packs or ice cubes in a plastic bag wrapped in a washcloth on top of it to decrease the inflammation and appease the pain for the first twenty-four hours only. After the twenty-four hours, apply hot water in a plastic bag tied up and wrapped in a washcloth. Both treatments must be applied every two hours for fifteen minutes only. It can be four to five times a day until there's no more pain and swelling because pain is usually caused by inflammation or swelling. The abscess may disappear also in two to three days or before. Nevertheless, continue to drink hot ginger tea to decrease swelling and spring water of eight eight-ounce cups per day to flush your system and lemonade from store with no artificial sweetener and chemicals or fresh home made only. Eat nutritious foods, fresh fruits and leafy vegetables, beans, nuts, fat-free dairy, whole-grain cereals and breads, brown rice, lean meat, poultry, and fish. Don't forget to be active, to breathe fresh oxygenated air to cleanse your system and prevent this type of abscess or any abscess from afflicting you.

ATHEROMATOUS ABSCESS

This is an abscess in the form of a softening in the wall of a blood vessel as a result of atherosclerosis. To prevent or alleviate the pain and cure this type of abscess, you have to be active, walk, stand up, or move around the best you can while having it. And when you don't make a schedule to exercise daily, while sitting or traveling by car or motorcycle, stop in rest areas every two hours and walk for ten minutes at your own pace. At home, while watching TV, stand up and walk every two hours during commercials or not to prevent clots and fat thrombus. Stay away from fatty saturated foods; hydrogenated, partially hydrogenated, or trans fat; vegetable oil; fast-food; fried food; and junk foods. Eat only food cooked with olive oil and canola oil or any other vegetable oil without hydrogen that makes it last longer, but can harm you. The good oils can decrease inflammation in your vessel wall. Decrease intake of dairy food and eat lean protein, plant protein, such as avocado, nuts, soy, and beans. Drink bottled spring water six to eight cups a day, 100 percent juices, citrus fruit and berries, white eggs any style except fried. All the above foods and drinks can decrease your LDL or fatty cholesterol and increase your HDL or good cholesterol, which in turn can fortify the soft wall and remove the plaques and decrease atherosclerosis.

AXILLARY ABSCESS

This is an abscess of the axilla or the armpit, which is on the outside of the body. This abscess is very uncomfortable because of the part of the body where it develops. But this abscess is less dangerous, easier to dissolve on its own, and less painful than many abscesses. To cure and prevent this abscess, leave this area very clean and dry at all times. Try to shave this area if you have a lot of hair in it, especially in the summertime. Don't use chemicals to shave it; use clean, sharp, and new disposable razor blades or electric shaver. Wash with clean warm water and mild liquid soap with no chemicals and no colors or scent and pat dry with soft tissue. Do not use deodorant or antiperspirant in that area during the abscess. At times when at home, leave your affected arm up to air for oxygen and hold next to a light from the room or from a lamp because this type of abscesses are caused by anaerobic bacteria toxin that don't like oxygen, light, and dryness. Adding all three of these factors to good nutrition with fresh fruits, citrus and berries, melons, tomato, green leafy vegetables, salads, whole-grain cereal, breads, beans, nuts, soy, lean protein, fat-free dairy, and olive oil, fish, and poultry can cure and prevent the reappearance of this type of abscess.

BARTHOLIN ABSCESS

This is an abscess of the Bartholin's gland. They are two small compound mucous glands situated on each side of the vaginal opening at the base of the labia major. They provide vaginal lubrication during coitus. This type of abscess are partly outside of the body and can be uncomfortable due to the location. When inflammation occurs, it can be painful.

Treatment

Wash with cool water running over the area with all-natural liquid mild soap. Do not touch the area, dry with patted tissue, leave legs open to air, oxygen, and light to prevent moisture, darkness, and lack of oxygen due to multiplication of anaerobic bacteria that are usually the cause of this type of abscesses. Prevent aggravation by abstaining from all activities in this area.

For fast healing and stopping reoccurrence of this type of abscesses, eat citrus fruits, berries, melons, tomato, flaxseed whole, whole-grain breads and cereals, pasta, brown rice, leafy vegetables, foods with antioxidants, omega-3 fatty acids, lycopene, low-fat or fat-free dairy, lean meat, lean poultry, and organic foods in general, naturally sweetened, chemical-free foods. Eat foods with vitamins A, C, B, D, and K and fiber. Eat nuts, seeds, dry prunes, dry apricots, pitted black olives in water, olive oil, red wine vinegar on romaine lettuce, carrots, avocado, dry beans and legumes. Decrease stress by using imagery, meditation, relaxation, rest, and laughter and walk when you can.

BLIND ABSCESS

A blind abscess is an abscess that gets no opening, for example, gum abscess, which we already covered as with alveolar abscess.

BICAMERAL ABSCESS

This abscess is like any other abscesses we had already covered except this abscess has two pockets instead of one unlike the others.

TREATMENT

Same as the others depending on where this abscess is situated, and nutrition is practically the same.

BILE DUCT ABSCESS

This is an abscess inside of the body in the bile duct, which is detected by medical tests and diagnosis by a physician. Symptoms are usually, fever, jaundice, loss of appetite, and pain due to inflammation. See your doctor immediately and continue food protection and infection control techniques, eat good nutritious foods itemized for other abscesses, and be active, decrease stress, sleep well, and rest.

BILHARZIASIS ABSCESS

This is an abscess in the intestinal wall caused by schistosoma. Schistosoma is a genus of blood flukes belonging to the family schistomatidae, class *trematoda. The adults live in the blood vessels of visceral organs. The eggs make their way into the bladder or intestines and are discharged in urine and feces. The eggs hatch into miracidia, which enter snails and transform into sporocysts. These develop into daughter sporocysts that give rise to fork-tailed cercacia. These leave the snails and enter the final host directly through the skin or through mucous membrane. To prevent this type of transferred infection, good hand washing, use of barrier to prevent contamination, infection control, good nutrition are a must.*

Nutrition

Eat fresh fruits and leafy vegetables, nuts, whole grain for folic acid, vitamin B12, and all the B-vitamin family, which are as follows: all orange colors of food, such carrots, cantaloupe, summer squash, apricot, sweet potato, oranges. Eat all citrus fruits for vitamin C and other fruits too like berries, pineapple, peaches, plums, nectarine, tangelo, kiwis, apple, pears, grapefruits. Eat food with vitamins A, E, and K. Eat fat-free or reduced-fat dairy such as cheese and yogurt and drink milk for protein and minerals. Eat lean protein meat, poultry and fish, and tofu and soy. Don't eat fried, fatty, and junk foods. Eat high-fiber foods, complex carbohydrates, whole-grain foods, dry beans, legumes, nuts, and dry prunes. Drink seven to eight eight-ounce cups of bottled spring water a day and 100 percent fruit juices only. Decrease stress, sleep seven to eight hours at night or daytime as needed, rest, laugh, dance, sing, party with friends and family, and exercise or walk daily.

BONE ABSCESS

An abscess of the bone, Brodie's abscess, was discovered by Sir Benjamin Collins Brodie, an English surgeon. They usually appear at the head of a bone, for example, head of the tibia. They are of tubercular origin from subacute staphylococcal infection. Symptoms are: aching pains followed by swelling and tenderness on movement. Symptoms are less acute but similar to osteomyelitis.

Treatment

Practice food protection, infection control, and good hygiene to fight the bacteria named staphylococci. Since this abscess is in the outside of the body where you can see and touch, keep area clean, exposed to light, dryness, and oxygen. Wash the area often with warm water, apply ice compress the first twenty-four hours for fifteen minutes every four hours. After twenty-four hours, apply warm compress as hot as you can stand it for another day the same way. Use barriers, gloves, to touch all contaminated equipment, linens, and other body parts. Since this one is from bacteria, you have to use precautions to prevent contamination of other people. Nutrition is like for all abscesses. Just follow what is already recommended for the other abscesses. The minor difference is that you need to eat foods that contain more minerals, such as calcium, potassium, iron, and magnesium to revitalize your bones.

BRAIN ABSCESS

Intracranial abscess is one that involves the brain or its membrane. It is seldom primary but usually occurs secondary to infection of the middle ear, nasal sinuses, face, or skull or from fractures. It may also have a metastatic origin arising from septic foci in the lungs (bronchiectasis, empyema, lung abscess) in bone (osteomyelitis) or heart (endocarditis). Infection of nervous tissue by the invading organism results in necrosis, liquefaction, and edema of surrounding tissues. Brain abscess may be acute, subacute, or chronic. Their clinical manifestations depend on part of the brain involved, size, virulence of infecting organisms, and other factors synonymous to cerebral and intracranial abscess.

Symptoms

Severe and persistent headache usually localized over infected area, fever, vomiting, vertigo, malaise, sometimes irritability, and other mental symptoms.

Treatment

Chemotherapy and surgical intervention may be required.

To prevent or go together with medical treatment and after to stop reoccurrence, good nutrition is the best. Eat organic and natural foods only. Drink bottled spring water and decrease food with chemicals. Eat everything fresh: fruits, vegetables, whole grains, and nuts. Avoid fast foods, preserved foods, processed foods, fatty food, fried foods, simple carbohydrates, bleached flour, artificial sweeteners, junk food, sugar, and sodium or table salt. Eat foods with omega 3 and 6 fatty acid, vitamin C, folic acid, ascorbic acid, and all the minerals needed for good nutrition. Boost your immune system with tea, mushrooms, onions, garlic, romaine lettuce, collard greens, kale, broccoli, ginger, cinnamon, thymes, cloves, flaxseed, sunflower seeds, and Echinacea.

BREAST ABSCESS

Abscess of the mammary gland that appears after giving birth to a child. These types of abscesses are usually due to lactation, engorgement of milk in the duct.

Prevention and Treatment

Let the baby suck to extract milk from the breast while feeding or if the baby is not breast-fed, extract milk with a pump artificially and get a prescription from your doctor to dry the milk. To treat this type of abscess, surgery may be necessary if the abscess is already fully developed. If the abscess has just started, with no swelling and no pain yet except a little discomfort to the site, just apply cold compress alternated by warm compress every two hours for fifteen minutes. Symptoms are usually fever, pain, and inflammation or swelling at the site. To stop reoccurrence, good nutrition with nonfat dairy products, fresh fruits and vegetables, and whole grains to make the milk flow normally is needed. Eat foods rich in calcium and other mineral and lean proteins. Avoid pungent, spicy foods like garlic, onion, basil, oregano, hot peppers, black pepper, and ginger that can repulse the baby and prevent sucking and lactation flow.

BURSAL ABSCESS

This is an abscess that occurs in the bursa tissue between the bones. Almost everything is the same as with the bone abscess except that instead of the head of the bones, this is the tissue between the bones and it's in the outside of the body where you can see, feel, and touch. In addition to elevating the part if they are legs and arms by placing them on top of a low table or bench or just a pillow or cushions, apply cold and warm compresses alternately every two hours for fifteen minutes each time. Nutrition: eat the same delicious, organic, and natural fruits, vegetables, whole-grain food, nuts, dry beans, lean proteins, and good oils, for example, olive, canola, and non hydrogenated or trans fat vegetable oils. Stay away from fatty foods, fried foods, and some chemicals, fat dairy and fat protein.

CIRCUMSCRIBED ABSCESS

Abscess limited or confined by surrounding tissue. If you can locate it, apply cold and warm compresses alternately every two hours for fifteen minutes. After twenty-four hours, change the cold compresses at first to warm compresses for another twenty-four hours every two hours for fifteen minutes. Drink ginger and cinnamon tea to decrease or prevent swelling and eat all the good foods that you already know by now. And stay away from the bad foods, which you know also. Exercise, walk, and move around. Do not sit or lie down for more than two hours straight unless it's bedtime.

CIRCUMTONSILLAR ABSCESS

This is an abscess around the tonsil in your throat. You can probably see it because the area seems bigger than usual and the normal pink color may change to red at the beginning and white and covered with mucous later on after inflammation. For pain, gargle warm saltwater, followed by eating ice cream, ice, and soft foods and no spicy food or hot drink to prevent irritation and aggravation. Apply ice pack on the outside by your neck. If you start treatment right away, it wouldn't last too long. But even after it's gone, see your doctor. To prevent, eat good foods rich in nutrients and vitamins that you need. Drink 100 percent fruit juice and spring water of eight eight-ounce cups per day to cleanse and flush out toxins.

DIFFUSE ABSCESS

This is a collection of pus not circumscribed by a well-defined capsule. This abscess can appear anywhere on the outside of the body. And by the time you notice it, it's already gone because it's usually the swelling that contain the pus that makes the abscess painful and noticeable. But if the pus is already showing and already out, the pressure is relieved. If you can see it, clean the area very well with warm water and liquid soap. Stay away from fatty foods and fast and fried foods. Eat only organic and nutritious foods that you already know from other abscesses.

DRY ABSCESS

Dry abscess is one that disappears without pointing or breaking, almost the same as the precedent except that this one doesn't even give you a chance to see it and do anything with it. By the time you notice the dry skin where it was, it's already gone. Keep good hygiene, eat good nutritious foods organic and natural, and drink a lot of bottled spring water.

EMBOLIC ABSCESS

Abscess due to a septic embolus, which is a mass of un-dissolved matter present in the blood or lymphatic vessel, brought there by blood or lymph current.

Treatment and Prevention

Practice food protection and infection control from the previous book T.H.A.T.S., The Health Assistance to Some.

Eat food that can boost your immune system to fight bacteria so they wouldn't get into your bloodstream and make you septic. Good organic and natural non processed foods can reduce or prevent this abscess. Eat garlic, all color s of onions, mushrooms, and fresh fruits for vitamin C, fat-free dairy for calcium and other minerals, lean proteins and plant protein, and all the rest of the good foods that you already know. Consult your doctor in case you need antibiotics. Keep elevated the part of the abscess that you can see and be active to prevent blood clot and promote oxygen-rich red blood cells.

EMPHYSEMATOUS ABSCESS

This is an abscess containing air or gas usually in the lungs; you can't see it but can feel pain and discomfort while breading. Consult your doctor, eat same good food, practice food protection, infection control, and exercise as much as you can to promote good air exchange of oxygen-rich blood cells and carbon dioxide. Good nutrition and exercises, like a walk in the morning, and vitamins needed go a long way with this abscess's cure and prevention.

ENDAMEBIC AMEBIC ABSCESS

Again, this abscess has to do with microorganism, parasites, and germs.

Good hygiene, practice of infection control and food protection in the previous book is a must. The rest is good nutrition; avoid processed food, fatty, and fast foods. Stay clean and dry, drink bottled spring water eight eight-ounce cups per day, and see your doctor if persistent.

FUNGAL ABSCESS

Again, this abscess is caused by fungus usually around the toenail.

Treatment

Apply white vinegar on a piece of cotton and let soak daily for a few minutes. Wash with warm water and liquid soap, keep dry and outside of shoes and socks when at rest at home as long as possible. Apply 70 percent rubbing alcohol patted dry, and bring a lamp close to the spot for fifteen minutes. When walking in public places such as the gym, wear flip-flop shoes to protect you from germs and fungus. Good hygiene, good nutrition, and vitamins are needed to prevent or solve this problem.

GAS ABSCESS

An abscess containing gas due to the presence of gas-forming organisms such as clostridium perfringen. This abscess can be in any part of the body. This organism is a genus of bacteria belonging to the family Bacillaceae. They are anaerobic, spore-forming rods and are widely distributed in nature; over 250 species are recognized. They are common in soil and in the intestinal tract of man and animals and are frequently found in wound infections. Several are pathogenic in man, being the primary causative agents of gas gangrene.

Prevention

Good hygiene, infection control, food protection practice, good nutrition, and activities that you already know from previous examples of abscesses can pull you through, cure you, and prevent this to happen.

GINGIVAL ABSCESS

An abscess of the gum is the same as the alveolar abscess with the difference that it can be in any part of the gum and not necessarily at the root of a tooth.

Treatment

Shake warm saltwater, apply hot compresses with a new clean washcloth and press it down as much as you can take it. If the swelling decreases, you wouldn't even have pain because the inflammation is what causes the pain. This type of abscess can even be dissolved before you even make it to the dentist. It would be good to see a dentist who wouldn't even see anything even with X-ray sometimes. The same good oral hygiene, good cleaning very often, good nutrition, food protection and infection control practice, and exercises can cure and prevent this type of abscesses.

HELMINTHIC ABSCESS

One due to the presence of parasitic worms. Good hand washing with warm water and liquid soap in a washbasin going to the sewer after using bathroom or anything dirty. Use barriers when touching your cooked or raw food to eat or to serve others. Practice infection control, food protection from previous book. And eat all the good foods in the previous example of abscesses plus papaya and drink hot ginger tea with cinnamon very often to treat, cure, and prevent reoccurrence of this abscess.

Hematic Abscess: abscess due to an extravagated blood clot.

Hemorrhagic Abscess: containing blood.

Hepatic Abscess: abscess of the liver, especially an amebic abscess caused by organisms.

Hot Abscess: is an acute abscess that is covered from the beginning of the abscess chapter.

Hypostatic Abscess is a wandering abscess.

Idiopathic abscess is due to unknown causes.

Iliac Abscess: an abscess in the iliac region, which is a bone abscess. Apply the same as for bone abscess already covered.

Intradural Abscess: one within the layers of the dura matter or tissue of the brain. Refer to brain abscess already covered.

Intracranial or brain or cerebral abscess also already covered.

Ischiorectal abscess in the ischiorectal fossa or rectum, also already covered.

Kidney abscess of the renal cortex is one on top of your kidney and inside of you. This one needs to be detected by medical tests or diagnosis by a physician. To prevent, ameliorate, and stop reoccurrence, practice food protection, infection control, good hygiene, eating of nutritious food and drinking a lot of bottled spring water, adding to your doctor's intervention.

LACRIMAL GLAND ABSCESS OR SUPPURATION

In lacrimal gland suppuration of the lacrimal gland in your eyes, wash with sterile water from drugstores, wash your hand before touching your eyes, practice infection control, food protection, and good hygiene. If the pus is already out, there is no pain. But it's good to see an eye doctor to prescribe eye drops with antibiotic. And the rest, you already know which is to eat all the good foods in previous examples plus carrots, eggs, almond and walnuts because they are good for your eyesight. Eggs have lutein, an antioxidant that protects your eyes from cataracts.

Almonds and walnuts are rich in omega-3 fatty acids; one or more servings will cut the risk of macular degeneration that causes blindness in adults. Six ounces of fatty fish, tuna, and salmon boost intake of omega-3 fatty acids. Broccoli protects your eyes from damage by the sun due to an antioxidant called sulforaphane. Broccoli sprouts have fifty times more sulforaphane than the mature plant.

From A to W, of the alphabet, there is the name of an abscess; most of the time the abscesses are the same with a different name. To complete this chapter on abscesses, let us talk about some skin interstitial abscesses caused by bacterial infections.

ABSCESSES CAUSED BY STAPH AUREUS

Staph aureus is a species commonly present on the skin and mucous membranes, especially those of the nose and mouth, characterized by production of a golden yellow pigment. They are cause of suppurative conditions, such as boils, carbuncle, and internal abscesses. The condition of staphylococcus aureus with metacillin resistant can turn to a deadly condition called MRSA.

For this type of abscesses, surgery, medical treatment, antibiotics, and sometimes contact isolation are emphasized or needed. Nevertheless, a good nutritious diet with low-fat, lean protein, green leafy vegetables, colorful vegetables, fruits and nuts, whole-grain foods, drinking a lot of bottled spring water, good hygiene can do the trick for this abscess too.

The bottom line for all abscesses is to have a good nutritious diet of fat-free dairy, lean meat, poultry, seafood, fish, and nuts, which are organic, all-natural, 100 percent fruit juices, spring bottled water, food protection. For information, refer to T.H.A.T.S., the previous book. Know about USDA, FDA, and expiration date in foods and read labels. Make sure that you eat foods that contain vitamins that you need.

Foods that contain Vitamin A and B complex are kale, collard greens, avocado.

Foods that contain vitamin C are broccoli, green pepper, most fruits; ascorbic acid can be obtained by eating pineapples.

Foods that contain bioflavonoids: broccoli, yogurt.

Foods that contain vitamin E: collard greens, swish chard, all green leafy vegetables.

Herbs: The ones that are good for reducing inflammation and swelling, cleansing, and speeding up healing are bromelain, cayenne, or capsicum, dandelion root or leaves, red cloves, yellow dock, chamomile, lemonade from fresh lemon, echinacea, soma, goldenseal tea, ginger, and cinnamon tea. Eat watermelon for skin abscesses because it contains linoleic acid. Eat cantaloupe for beta-carotene and summer squash for vitamins A, B, and D. Eat celery, romaine lettuce, green leafy vegetables, and all in the cabbage family.

ACIDOSIS

This is the excessive acidity of body fluids due to an accumulation of acids as in diabetic acidosis, or renal disease, or an excessive loss of bicarbonate as in a renal disease. The hydrogen ion concentration is increased and thus the pH is decreased; as a result, you have a fluid and electrolyte imbalance.

1. Carbon dioxide - Acidosis resulting from CO_2 retention as in drowning or decreased respiration or gaseous.
2. Compensated - Acidosis in which the pH of body fluids has been returned to normal. Compensatory mechanisms maintain the normal ratio of bicarbonate to carbonic acid in blood plasma although the bicarbonate level is decreased.
3. Diabetic - Acidosis occurring in advanced stages of uncontrolled diabetes mellitus due to accumulation of ketone bodies, which can cause diabetic coma.
4. Metabolic - Acidosis resulting from increase in acids other than carbonic acid. Possible causes are excessive ingestion of acids or acid salts, ketosis, renal disease, impaired liver function.
5. Renal - Acidosis due to impaired kidney function. The acidosis is induced by excessive loss of bicarbonate or the inability to excrete phosphoric and sulfuric acids.
6. Respiratory - Acidosis secondary to pulmonary insufficiency resulting in retention of carbon dioxide.
7. Acids poisoning - Ingestion of a toxic acid. Treatment: dilute with large amount of water, given orally, milk, egg white, magnesium oxide, milk of magnesium, lime water, and aluminum hydroxide gel. Avoid carbonates as neutralizers because in the presence of strong acids, they react to produce carbon dioxide gas. This may cause distention and rupture of the stomach. In a case like this,

people should go to the emergency room to receive demulcents and morphine for pain. The use of emetics and stomach tubes is dangerous.

Again, acidosis is a condition that causes the body chemistry to be imbalanced and overly acidic. If you read the first book T.H.A.T.S., The Health Assistance to Some, *which covers acid alkali and the pH balance of fluids and electrolytes, especially in blood in food protection program, you won't be surprised at all of acidosis condition. In the previous book, there is an anagram called FAT TOM, which the letter F is for "foods," the letter A is for "acid" and "alkali," the first letter T for "temperature" for foods to be safe, the second letter T is for "time" in dealing with food. The letter O is for "oxygen" or air that gets to do with bacteria in foods, which can be aerobic or anaerobic, gram negative or positive. The aerobic bacteria like air or oxygen in the air. And anaerobic bacteria don't like air or oxygen in the air. Gram-positive bacteria are shaped like grapes in a bunch. Gram-negative bacteria are shaped like rods. The letter M is for "moisture" that keeps bacteria alive and awake that we don't need in and around our foods cooked or raw sometimes.*

The reason I explain the above is in case the readers of this book hadn't read the first book, which detailed food protection and infection control, but not the diseases and foods causing them or curing them and preventing them.

Here are some signs and symptoms of acidosis: insomnia, sighing very often, retaining water, recessed eyes, arthritis pain, migraine headaches, abnormal and too low blood pressure, acidic and strong perspiration, dry, hard rock-like stools, foul-smelling stools accompanied by burning sensation in the anus, alternating constipation and diarrhea, difficulty swallowing, bad breath or halitosis, burning sensation in the mouth and under the tongue, sensitivity of the teeth to vinaigrette, salad dressing, citrus fruits, or other acidic fruits, bumps on the tongue or roof of the mouth. Sometimes frequent belching, burping occurs.

CLASSIFICATIONS

There are two classifications of acidosis: respiratory and metabolic. The respiratory acidosis is caused by an interruption of the acid control of the body, resulting in overabundance of the acidic fluids or the decrease of alkali or base. This happens if the lungs are unable to remove carbon dioxide. Respiratory acidosis can be caused by asthma, bronchitis, obstruction of airway or passage. Respiratory acidosis are sometimes mild or severe. It all depends on what precipitates it.

Metabolic Acidosis

Metabolic acidosis occurs when chemical changes in the body disturb the body's acid alkali of the blood pH or fluids and electrolyte balance. At the beginning of this chapter, some medical conditions that can cause acidosis were mentioned.

Other factors or situations can cause acidosis too. They are taking aspirin in large quantities, seasoning your foods, meat, poultry, fish, seafood, and other foods with too much vinegar, lemon juice, lime juice, orange juice; drinking too much citrus fruit juice, eating too much acidic foods, eating improper diet, malnutrition, obesity, ketosis, being angry, argumentative, stressed out, anorexia, toxemia, high anxiety, fear, high fever, taking too much vitamins and supplements, especially niacin and vitamin C.

Acid-Forming Foods

Alcohol is the number one because it's made from acidic fruits and vegetables when they change to acid. Therefore, use any alcohol with moderation, which is also in the first book.

Asparagus, beans if the starch is left in after cooking. Soak beans overnight to get most of the starch and the sugar out.

Brussels sprouts, catsup, coffee, cornstarch, cranberries, mustard, olives in vinegar, pasta. Wash pasta in cold water to get the starch out from colander. Pepper of all colors, plums, prunes, sauerkraut, soft drinks, food with vinegar added to them, foods with sugar added to them and vinegar are to stay away from if you have the tendency to be acidic or have acidosis. Smoking can cause acidosis too. A great number of drugs are acidic or acid forming, except the antacids. When taking medication, ask your pharmacist about acidosis and the drug that you are taking for contraindication or untoward side effects.

Some foods with some acid-forming quality that are not too much: cheeses, butter, coconut, some grains, ice cream, ice milk, nuts, and seeds.

For this reason, you can't eat too much of any one type of foods. You need to eat a little of each group of food to balance your diet and provide you with all the vitamins, nutrients, and minerals that your body needs to be healthy.

ACNE

Acne is an inflammatory disease of the sebaceous glands and hair follicles of the skin characterized by comedones, papules, and nodules. Scarring is common and dangerous in black people or mixed Spanish or mixed black with white due to an incurable condition of the skin called keloid or a bumpy discolored scar formation. They usually get bigger with surgery or injection and dry-ice application. The more you treat them, the bigger they get. If you don't touch them or bother them, they sometimes get smaller or erased completely as time goes by. But if on the contrary you listen to people that think they are cancers and urge you to see a doctor that treat them in any way they know, they can become real big and ugly, shiny, reddish, pale whitish in color depending on the person's complexion. They are not dangerous because they don't cause death. They are bad for two reasons: disfiguration and if on top of a major organ or blood vessel where they can nourish and get bigger or develop their own blood vessels. Otherwise, they are usually benign (not malignant).

Example

Some people suffer from keloids badly for some time. People have them from vaccination as a child, and doctors from Europe, especially France, usually tell the parents not to touch them. But people in United States don't know about this disease or skin condition. When these people wear sleeveless or spaghetti-strap dresses, some people start to bother them with their concern and urge them to see a doctor for skin cancer. The keloids on some children are the size of a grape seed for many years. After the people with keloids listen to people without knowledge of this skin condition, they would go see some doctors who burn them with dry ice, turn them to the size of a plum, and then flatten them to a charcoal barbeque sausage. When these people start with treatment, after each one, they most of the time find themselves in the emergency room in excruciating pain. Some people try every kind of treatment. They have them cut, injected with steroid that make them bigger, cortisone, and other drugs, which make them itch in the summer and winter. People need to notice that most people like to give advice about something that they don't know. And they don't believe you either because they think that they know so much that it's you that doesn't know. Sometimes it's not so much because they care but because they want to prove their expertise, which can be erroneous. Other times you may notice keloids in people's ears after they pierce the lobe and in some men's chin and the back of the neck from shaving or haircut. People also can get keloids from cuts, bruises, surgery, and especially children from hurting and scrapping their skin from playing.

Other times it can be a keloid formed from an injection side such as the forearm in receiving PPD test or vaccine against tuberculosis. Unfortunately for this child or person, after a few years, a keloid is developed from the site. By the time the same person has to take another PPD as a job requirement, the person giving the test notices the keloid and asks, "What is this?" He gets the answer, "It's a PPD I received two years ago that developed a keloid." The person questioning answers, "Keloid, a skin disease, I never heard of it!" That's all you need to have a PPD positive on your record for life and having to take a chest X-ray every medical place you go. Sometimes, besides the chest X-ray you are given antibiotic needlessly and get reported to the health department as a "protocol." This is the most cruel label and torture that one has to go through from a bunch of ignorant people. What don't people inquire and search and learn. Some French doctors just look and say, "Ha, you form keloids! No need to give this person a PPD test, this is not a positive result." Some people are just followers who repeat or do things without questioning like they don't have a mind of their own. Some children are better than them because when adults give them an answer that they are not satisfied of, they ask, "How come?" until you give them the satisfactory answers.

Acne is an inflammatory skin disorder characterized by pimples, blackheads, and whiteheads. To some degree, it affects about 80 percent of all Americans between the ages of ten to fifty years old. According to the American Academy of Dermatology and other studies, acne has become the most commonly treated skin abnormality. It looks to me that modern lifestyles contribute to this change in statistics. For acne sufferers, it's not just a cosmetic problem. Some of the consequences are emotional, mental stress, and low self-esteem and self-confidence.

Acne often appears at puberty when the body dramatically increases its production of androgen male sex hormones. These hormones stimulate the production of keratin, a type of protein, and sebum, an oily skin lubricant. If sebum is secreted faster than it can move through the pores, a blemish arises. The excess oil makes the pores sticky, allowing bacteria to become trapped inside instead of coming out from the cells through the pores or holes in the skin.

Blackheads form when sebum combines with skin pigments and plugs the holes or pores. If the scales below the surface of the skin become filled with sebum, whiteheads appear. In severe cases, whiteheads build up, spread under the skin, and rupture, which eventually spreads the inflammation. Proper skin care is important in treatment and prevention of acne. Acne is not cause by uncleanness alone, but also as a result of overactive oil glands.

Although more than 20 million teenagers suffer from this condition, acne is not just affecting kids anymore. It is also affecting a large number of adults even older up to fifty years old and children younger than twelve to ten years old. Teenage acne commonly occurs on the face and upper torso or body. Adult acne occurs only on the chin and jaw. They are fewer but with more painful blemishes or discoloration.

Some women suffer premenstrual acne flare-ups due to the release of progesterone after ovulation. Oral contraceptives loaded with progesterone can cause breakouts of acne also. The presence of candidiasis can also cause hormonal changes that cause the liver to produce the wrong substances for healthy sebum. Candidiasis caused by candida albicans, which is a single-celled fungus, always present in the genital and intestinal tracts, can cause acne. When we get to the disease candidiasis, we will talk some more about it. For now let's stay on acne.

FACTORS

Factors that can contribute to acne are the following:

1. *Heredity or genetic makeup.*
2. *Oily skin.*
3. *Hormone.*
4. *Menstrual cycles.*
5. *Allergies.*
6. *Stress.*
7. *Use of some types of drugs, such as steroids, lithium, oral contraceptives, antiepileptic drugs.*
8. *Malnutrition and vitamin or mineral deficiencies.*
9. *Exposure to industrial pollutants such as machine oils, coal tar derivatives, battery acid, chlorinated hydrocarbons, swimming in inadequately clean and sanitized pools. All can cause acne.*
10. *A body pH blood and pH fluids and electrolytes imbalance with too much acid or acidic or too much alkaline or alkalosis can cause acne.*
11. *Bacteria in the skin can cause acne.*

SKIN

Let us talk about the skin. The skin is the largest organ in the body. One of the skin functions is to eliminate toxin or a portion of the body's toxic waste products through sweating. When the body contains more toxins than the kidneys and liver can effectively discharge, the skin takes over the job. As more and more toxins get out of the skin, the less healthy the skin becomes.

The skin needs to breathe, and if the pores or holes in the skin become clogged, the germs that cause acne multiply and thrive because they are protected against sunshine and oxygen in the air; then acne will become more severe. Dirt, dust, oils, pollution, and chemicals can clog the pores also. Nevertheless, this problem can be eliminated, treated, and prevented with treatment, good nutrition, proper care, and things to stay away from.

TREATMENT

The skin can be properly cleaned by using an alcohol swab or some cotton balls soaked in 70 percent rubbing alcohol or witch hazel formula, astringent cleanser, to clean the skin of the face, neck, and all the affected parts of the body before everyday washing. With a natural soap free from chemicals, no dye, no scent or fragrance free, and warm water, thoroughly wash your face, neck, and all other parts you want to treat or prevent from acne. You can use a clean washcloth or your bare hands to take out the sebum or oil and everything else. Next, rinse with cool or cold water and pat dry with tissue or clean towels. Because of this knowledge dated in childhood, I never had acne, and no one in my family ever had acne either. At least for this time and this condition, they listened to me and did the same thing. Use only water-based, natural, organic, chemical-free, and unscented cosmetics.

Adding to the proper cleaning and daily washing, good nutrition and exercise or activity, and not being overweight can prevent and cure acne. In mild to moderate cases of acne, no need to see a dermatologist or apply prescription drugs.

NUTRITION

Foods, drugs, supplements, and food additives or chemicals to stay away from: fat foods, saturated animal fats, vegetable oil with trans fat, partially hydrogenated fats, hydrogenated fats, processed foods, salty food, concentrated sugary foods, fried foods, fast-foods, junk foods, smoked foods and some foods that contain certain additives and chemicals. Stay away from poorly or uncooked foods, foods contaminated with bacteria, mold, and fungus.

Alcohol, Nutrients and Drugs

Stop smoking cigarettes and cigars.

Alcohol should be consumed moderately, such as two ounces of hard liquor, one eight-ounce beer daily, one glass of four-ounce wine daily for women, a maximum. Otherwise, only two to three times a week is the ideal. For men, two drinks a day or sparingly should be the ideal.

Avoid kelp supplements and iodized salt.

Find out from your doctors about your prescription drugs or over-the-counter drugs to see if they are contraindicated to acne conditions.

NUTRITIOUS FOOD TO EAT

Eat foods from all the food groups starting with the starchy simple carbohydrates sparingly and complex carbohydrates: whole grains, breads, cereals, oats, bran, rice of all colors except white not too much, millet, barley, dried beans, peas, lentils, potato mostly sweet or yam, and whole-grain pasta. They contain zinc, a mineral good for healthy skin. Eat all fruits and vegetables fresh from produce department. Fruits and vegetables contain vitamins A and C. Eat foods with all the vitamins Bs also. To make sure that you have all the vitamins and minerals that you need, eat all colors of foods. By doing this, you can consume antioxidants, omega-3 fatty acids, and all vitamins in food and enzymes, hormones, and proteins. Eat lean proteins, meat, poultry, fish, and fat-free or low-fat dairy products in moderation.

ADRENAL CONDITIONS OR DISORDERS

Let us talk about the adrenal glands, which are a pair of triangular-shaped organs or glands that rest on top of the kidneys. Each gland normally weighs about five grams or a little less than one-fifth of an ounce. The gland is composed of two parts. The cortex or the outer section is responsible for the production of the hormones cortisone, cortisol, aldosterone, androstenedione, and dehydroepiandrosterone (DHEA). The medulla, or central section, secretes another hormone, adrenaline, also called epinephrine and norepinephrine, which functions as both a hormone and a neurotransmitter.

The adrenaline, cortisol, DHEA, and norepinephrine are the body's major stress hormones. The highest levels of these hormones are released in the morning and the lowest at night. Cortisol is also involved in the metabolism of carbohydrates and the regulation of blood sugar. Aldosterone helps to maintain electrolytes, for example, salt and water balance in the body. Androstenedione and DHEA are androgens and hormones that are similar to and can be converted as a cure-all for aging. However, very little is known about the action of DHEA in the body. And while it is available from numerous sources, it is also a steroidal hormone. DHEA is a steroidal hormone and should be used with caution by a doctor or a nurse under a doctor's supervision. The long-term effects of using DHEA are unknown. Adrenaline speeds up the rate of metabolism and produces other physiologic changes designed to help the body cope with danger. Adrenaline is produced when the body is under stress. Under circumstances of extreme stress, large amounts of cortisol are released also, which can lead to a host of health problems.

Some disorders that are directly related to the adrenal glands include reduced function usually referred to as low adrenal reserve. The adrenals still produce enough hormones to maintain a relatively normal state of health, but stressful situations increase the need for hormones that the malfunctioning adrenals can't produce, leading to anything from fatigue to total collapse. Symptoms of reduced adrenal function can include weakness, lethargy, fatigue, recurrent infections, dizziness, low blood pressure when standing, headaches, memory problems, food cravings, allergies, and blood sugar disorders.

ADDISON'S DISEASE

Addison's disease is a rare condition that develops if the adrenal cortex is seriously underactive. Remember, the adrenal glands are a pair of triangular-shaped organs or glands that rest on top of the kidneys and are composed of two parts that are the cortex and the medulla. As mentioned previously, the cortex or outer part of the glands is responsible for the hormones cortisone, cortisol, aldosterone, etc. The symptoms of Addison's disease include fatigue, loss of appetite, dizziness or fainting, low blood pressure, nausea, diarrhea, depression, craving salty foods, moodiness, decrease in the amount of body hair, and inability to cope with stress. In certain cases, the "fight or flight" is in application.

People affected by this disease may also constantly complain of feeling cold. Discoloration and darkening of the skin is common in people with this disease; discoloration of the knees, elbows, scars, skin folds, and creases in the palms are more noticeable when these body parts are exposed to the sun. The mouth, the vagina, and freckles, if any, may appear darker. This disease is also characterized by the development of bands of pigment running the length of the nails and darkening of the hair. The most common type of this disorder is the autoimmune Addison's disease. This appears when the immune system mistakenly attacks the tissue of the adrenal glands and destroys them. Other diseases associated with autoimmunity that affect *other endocrine glands are hypothyroidism, Schmidt's syndrome, insulin-dependent diabetes mellitus, and pernicious anemia. We talk about these diseases in other chapters or sections of the book according to the alphabetical list. Let's continue with Addison's disease, which requires lifelong treatment. Fortunately, people with Addison's disease can have a normal life expectancy if they stay on the proper medication as prescribed by their endocrinologist, which is a doctor or specialist in hormonal diseases.*

Treatment

Follow a very good diet, which is a lifestyle change with foods that contain Vitamin B complex, extra pantothenic acid vitamin B5, vitamin C with bioflavonoids, and coenzyme A. Use foods with all the minerals calcium; magnesium; beta-carotene from natural orange-colored fruits and vegetables; copper from nuts; potassium from nuts, bananas, oranges, potatoes; iron from calf liver sautéed in olive oil; and B vitamins and enzymes.

Activity

Get moderate exercises or just walk for a half hour daily or four to five days a week at your own pace first and progress later on. Be moderately active by doing yoga, belly dancing, or other fun and pleasurable activity that can release stress as much as possible. Go on vacations to the islands, enjoy the beach, the ocean, nature and sleep well for a good eight hours at night.

Nutrition

Eat a lot of fresh fruits and vegetables of all colors, especially the green leafy vegetables (four to five servings a day). Eat brewer's yeast white rice, legumes, beans, nuts, olive oil, and safflower oils, seeds, wheat germ, and whole grains. For protein, eat deep-water ocean fish, salmon and tuna (fresh ones cooked by you) at least three to four times a week. Use garlic, onions, mushrooms, pearl barley, and oats. These foods contain germanium, which is a very powerful stimulant of the immune system.

Foods to Stay Away from or Avoid

Avoid alcohol, caffeine, and tobacco because they are toxic to the adrenal glands. Stay away from fats, fried foods, ham, pork, processed foods, red meats, sodas, white sugar, and artificial sweeteners and white flour. These foods put a lot of stress on the adrenal glands.

AGING/AGE SPOTS

Let's talk about age spots, which are part of aging. Age spots are flat brown or beige, depending on the skin complexion. They can appear almost anywhere on the body as the person gets old or aged. Sometimes they are referred to as liver spots. Most of them appear on the face, neck, and hands. These brown spots are usually harmless. But they can be the sign of more serious underlying problems. They are the result of a buildup of waste products known as lipofuscin accumulation, a by-product of free radical damage in the skin cells. The liver spots are actually signs that the cells are full of the type of accumulated wastes that slowly destroy the body's cells, including brain and liver cells. The liver spots are the surface sign of free radical intoxication of the body that may affect internal structure as well, including the heart muscle and the retina in the eyes.

What makes the age spots happen are bad diet or just eating the wrong foods that are poor in vitamins and natural nutrients, consuming oxidized oils for a long time, fried foods, saturated fat foods, and fatty animal protein. Exposure to the sun too much can cause the development of free radicals that can damage the skin also. People who live in sunny climates and are constantly exposed to the sun have the most liver spots, per the color of their skin.

Lipofuscin formation is due to a deficiency of some important nutrients, vitamins, and minerals such as selenium, glutathione, chromium, dimethyl aminoethanol, and vitamins E. Smoking and consuming too much alcohol can increase production of lipofuscin that can damage the skin and other organs in the body.

AGING

Aging is a natural process. Aging is neither a disease nor a condition. If people know how to eat, what to eat, when to eat; what type of foods to eat for health; how to exercise, what type of exercise and activities to do, and when to do them; how to have fun; how to treat each other around them; what kind of social life to have; how to have a structured and organized lifestyle; how to be honest, clean inside and outside including their mind, actions, and soul; how to have integrity, they would age gracefully and look twenty or more years younger than their biological and chronological age.

The chronological age is just a number. But unfortunately in some civilizations, no matter how young you look, how strong, energetic, fast, brainy, fit, confident, happy, and all the attributes of youth you may have or feel, as soon as some people see your chronological age on a piece of paper, you are discarded in a trash bin or a far corner. As you turn in the late fifties going on sixty years old, you start having ads for wheelchairs, hearing aids, long-term care insurance, assisted living residence, cemetery plots, and everything that gets to do with old people. In some civilizations, old people are respected and admired for their wisdom, experience in life, acquired knowledge, and accomplishments. But in civilizations where people go by the norm, there is no exception and no one is unique. People are just a number in everything at any age including being old. And for not looking old, some people go through a lot of miseries for nothing because what counts in this type of civilization is the numbers.

What some people think about aging or their philosophies of what make people age are as follows:

The DNA Theory

The DNA in our bodies contains a genetic blueprint, which we inherit from our parents and ancestors. This is a unique code that determines numerous factors affecting aging. Things that happen during our lifetime that damage the DNA, such as exposure to pollutants, toxin, radiation, our diet, environmental factors, and lifestyle can affect the ability of our body to repair damage. This genetic damage can cause the production of abnormal protein and sugar protein complexes, which leads to defective cell repair, loss of cell elasticity, and other symptoms of the aging process.

The Neuroendocrine Theory

The pituitary gland and hypothalamus in the brain regulate the release of key hormones to influence cell metabolism, protein synthesis, immune functioning of all bodily cells. The theory is that the hypothalamus, over a period of time, loses its ability to regulate all these functions. The secretion of hormones gradually decreases, and hormone production process leads to aging. As a result, the decline in the polypeptide hormone insulin like growth factor 1, or IGF-1, is linked to a decline in cell activity. IGF-1 is a liver-produced product of human growth factor HGH, which is secreted by the pituitary. Research has shown that IGF-1 increases insulin sensitivity, increases lean body mass, reduces fat, and builds bone, muscle, and nerves. The IGF-1 has the ability to repair peripheral nerve tissue that has been damaged.

Free Radical or Oxidation Theory

This theory explains that unrepaired cumulative cell damage caused by free radicals, generated by normal metabolism and contributed to outside sources, is the cause for aging. Outside factors in the environment— for example, exposure to toxins, pollutants, radiation, alcohol, tobacco, and diet—cause highly reactive cell by-products called free radicals to be formed. These free radicals are molecules or portions of them that are capable of existing independently because they have odd numbers of electrons while normal electrons occur in pairs. Therefore, these electrons are unstable and react quickly with other compounds, trying to capture another needed electron to gain stability. As a result, an attacked molecule loses an electron to a free radical and becomes a free radical itself. Also in aging, there are oxygen-free radicals that take away an electron from another molecule to pair with their single free electrons. This process is called oxidation and can precipitate aging due to toxic metabolites accumulation and interfere with the function of cell membranes, protein synthesis, and cellular DNA/RNA.

As a result, cell energy production is wrongly affected and causes a faster aging process.

Cross-Linking Theory

According to scientists, when we have a normal metabolism, some sugars like glucose, fructose, and reactive compounds named aldehydes and ketones can attach to free amino groups on proteins. The result is a process called glycation and the protein is saddled with sugar molecules. Thus, this protein can react or cross-link with other proteins to cause a bond between the two. The resulting carbonyl group acts as a glue to attach the two proteins. Carbonyls are formed when either as a free radical or an aldehyde or a ketone reacts with amino acids on a protein. There is a possibility to have not just a protein to protein cross-linking, but also to lipid and protein to DNA cross-linking caused by large aggregates of damaged proteins around the tissues called advanced glycosylation end products. The end products can go on to react with free radicals to cause tissue damage through oxidation. They can also become mutagenic, cancer, causing and stimulating cells to produce more damaging free radicals. These products also act to accelerate a cell's death, a treatment to prevent, stop, inhibit cross-linking and reverse if not too late, the process of aging. This good news should be a must and a plus to all of us.

Immune Theory

Of course, the immune system slowly but surely becomes less effective as we get old. The thymus gland responsible for the production of thymic lymphoid or T-cells can decrease its function by up to 80 percent as we reach middle years. As we age, the immune system is less able to produce the antibodies, macrophages or natural killer cells and others that our body needs to fight off infections and other assaults from outside. Also there is a tendency to produce antibodies against the body itself, or the autoimmune response, which is responsible for a cohort of autoimmune diseases.

Telomere Theory

The cells of the body are replaced by means of cell division, and there is a limit on the number of times they may divide successfully. That is, most cells normally divide approximately fifty times before they stop dividing and die a natural death. It is theorized that the mechanism that controls cell division lies with the telomere, which is a cap-like structure on the end of each of the twenty-three pairs of chromosomes. Chromosomes are the helical structures of DNA that carry our genetic codes. Every time a cell divides, the telomere shortens up a bit. This constant shortening of the telomere means that after a certain number of divisions, the telomere disappears and the end of the chromosome begins to fray and stop dividing. This leads eventually to the death of the cell. Over a period of time, this cumulative cell death leads to aging. But an enzyme called telomerase has been discovered. This enzyme acts to repair damage to the telomeres and helps maintain their length and stability. The theory is that by using telomerase, we may be able to prolong cell life and slow down or even reverse the aging process.

Stem Cell Theory

This theory says that as we age, we begin losing stem cells from the reserve we had at birth. This means that our body's ability to repair and generate tissue is diminished and we accumulate more dysfunctional cells as time passes. Aging is simply the accumulation of the dysfunctional cells and the damage they cause to the skin, organs, the immune system, the muscles and every other system in our body can only be undone by addition of new stem cells.

Cell Metabolic Theory

This theory has a lot to do with nutrition. It says that good nutrition with foods rich in vitamins, minerals, and enzymes can slow down the aging process while caloric restriction can increase lifespan by affecting the cell division rate. Caloric restriction slowed down the aging process by an associated decrease in oxygen-free radicals produced by the mitochondria, which are the energy-generating structures in the cells (the powerhouse of cells). All the above are conceived according to some studies on animals. I am not aware of any study done on humans up to 2010 on physical and biological areas. Again, to clarify this statement, there may be some studies done successfully in this area that I don't know about. So feel free to research and investigate on your own. I heard, observed some cultural anthropological information, read about, and watched on TV some documentations about some parts of the world including the United States where people beat the aging process by many years and increase their lifespan up to past one hundred years old by consuming less calories than other people.

Psychology of Aging

I can't begin to explain how to fight aging without quoting Erik Erikson, my favored psychologist. Since I learned how to read, I had never spent one day of my life without thinking of Erikson's eight stages of development. In my early childhood, I went to a place named the French Quarter or Quartier Latin (French) from my country of birth, which was occupied by the French. There I bought with my own money earned from babysitting jobs a psychology book, and I learned about Erik Erikson. Since then and up to now, when I see an infant with a parent, a child, a teenager, a young adult, a middle-aged person, an elderly, or a person in the last stage or eighth stage of development, later adulthood which we need to talk about now, I think about Erikson.

According to Erikson and many other psychologists in nature versus nurture, there are too many changes that people must adjust to. These changes begin to interfere with activities of daily living. We can't afford to wait for old age to deal with these problems. To me, it is imperative to start early to solve some of them. Otherwise, it will be too late. Therefore, starting from adulthood, eighteen to forty years of age, we need to acquire knowledge on how to prepare aging. Aging will happen anyway. But we can prevent the deterioration, delay some of the ravaging and obvious symptoms, give ourselves a few more years of youth, fight the aging process for not starting too soon and cripple us.

According to Erik Erikson's eight stages of development, we have to resolve the conflict of this stage, which is ego integrity versus despair. The description of this stage is the following: Adults eventually review their lives. A life well spent result in a sense of well-being and integrity. Erikson would not expect that conflicts can be fully resolved. He said, "During old age, the life crisis involves integrity and despair. How could anybody have integrity and not also despair about certain things in his/her own life, about the human condition?" That was an idea about some aspects on preparing, delaying, and preventing premature aging besides eating good foods. You can refer to the previous book T.H.A.T.S., The Health Assistance to Some *for a lot of information about preventing aging.*

FIGHTING AGING AND WINNING

If you don't know what to eat, what good habits, scientific techniques, exercises, and activities to practice, after you pass forty years old, your body is going to change very fast on you. If you don't know good strategies to fight fat accumulation in your body, you are going to have bulges everywhere and even be obese before you even notice it. The bulges will be in places such as protruded abdomen, saggy breasts hanging down on top of your stomach all the way down to your belly, bags hanging down in your forearms, saddlebags by your hips and your behind down to your legs. Adding to the hanging fats and loose skin, you probably will start with varicose veins in your thighs and legs, facial hair, gray dull hair on your head, losing hair in your head first on your forehead, each side of your face, next thinning of your hair on your head with some bald spots in any place of your head. By your neck, your cheeks and your jaws, loose skin and wrinkles will definitely start before you know it, especially if you are under a lot of stress. Don't laugh! This picture is not funny although a good laugh is always welcome, but this time it's not.

Don't despair because if you know what good foods to eat, bad foods to stay away from, exercises and activities to enjoy, what kind of socialization to be involved in, what type of reading and writing to practice, what kind of knowledge to acquire, technique, table games, puzzles, mind tweezers and quizzes to do or take part of and enjoy, and how to decrease stress, you definitely will be able to delay aging, fight aging, prevent aging, save a few more years of youth, live longer, be healthier, look younger than you can even imagine. The way to do all the above is in this book and the previous book T.H.A.T.S., The Health Assistance to Some *will help you a great deal if you read it too.*

Let's start with certain foods that I have been researching, experimenting with, and using in daily diets that haven't let me down so far. Other people that I know have been using some of these foods with good results also and look ten to twenty years younger than their chronological age without plastic surgery or Botox injections.

WALNUT

Eat walnuts every day, at least eight whole or sixteen halves raw that you can shell or were already shelled for you at the baking goods section in any supermarket. Why? Because they are a great source of omega-3 acids that can make you feel full for a long time. This fact alone can make you lose weight or prevent you from gaining weight. Just know that weight can be a factor in aging.

WATER

To protect you from infections, boost your immune system, drink seven to eight cups of eight-ounce water daily before in between and after meals and snacks. Just add a drop of fresh lemon juice to your water. If you have a lot of pounds to lose, this will do the trick for you.

CINNAMON

Don't use sugar and artificial sweets to trick your brain because it wouldn't work. I know some women who drink diet sodas and juices, use artificial sweets in their coffee and tea all the time, but are as big as an elephant. It's better to use cinnamon for taste or just a little dark brown sugar in your drinks until you become used to no sugar or sweet at all. Cinnamon is not just for flavor when you put it in your drinks; sprinkle it on top of your dessert, or boil it and make your coffee, tea, or hot chocolate. This fact will help you to burn the fat, decrease swelling, decrease your fatty cholesterol (LDL), decrease your glucose or sugar level in your blood if you are a type 2 diabetic. It will thin your blood if you form clots or have deep-vein thrombosis. If you don't have these conditions yet, it will prevent you from having them and stay young for a lot of more years to come. Remember, cinnamon is good for a lot of other diseases that we will talk about alphabetically besides being a calories burner and calories free.

SALMON

Eat salmon for it has important minerals that all people need, but which older people need more. People over fifty years going seventy and older, especially women after menopause, need these minerals and vitamins because they help the hormone leptin to regulate their appetite. The most important vitamin is Vitamin D and the mineral is calcium.

HOT PEPPERS

Everybody should eat hot peppers unless it's not recommended for them due to certain conditions. Otherwise, eat hot pepper in your chili or salad and put hot sauce in most of your meals. Hot peppers burn fat. Therefore, the body can't store calories. Hot peppers contain a substance called capsaicin that makes it taste hot, heat up and melt the fat, clear insulin from the bloodstream before the fat can turn solid and accumulate.

FLAXSEED

Flaxseed ground or oil is high in fiber. It keeps you full for a long time, cuts your appetite, regulate your blood sugar or glucose so you don't need to eat all day all the bad foods high in calories that can make you fat and look old. Being fat and obese make people look older than they are biologically.

MORE GOOD FOODS TO PREVENT AGING

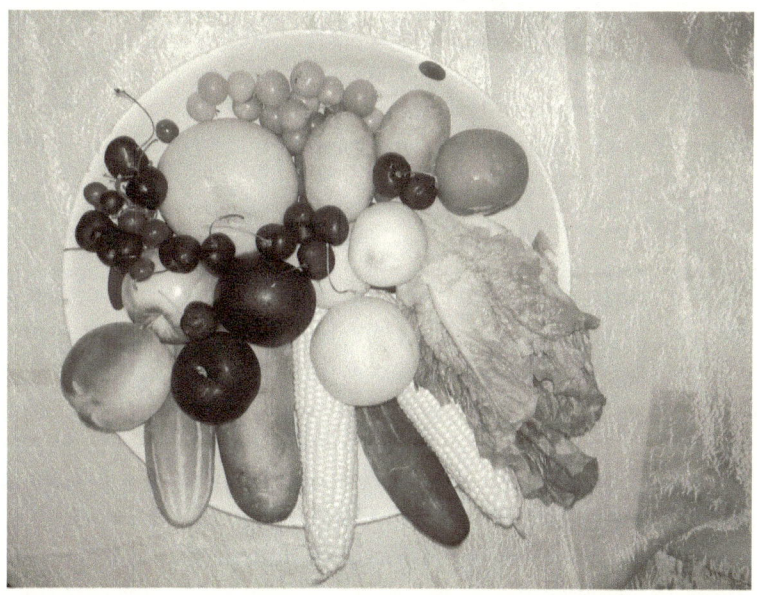

You can go back on time for ten to twenty years and even more. You can move the time machine or the hand of your biological clock several years back and reclaim the vitality of youth, the wide sunshine smile with glittering white teeth, your glowing elastic facial muscles, and shiny and full skin, and the ironic joyful twinkles in your eyes just by eating some wonderful miracle foods.

You don't have to sacrifice the snacks, desserts, and any food you like. Just add these foods in your diet or your daily eating if they are not already there. If you consume some of these foods daily, you don't have to open a bottle of vitamins and supplements unless you want to, which can be overdoing it, for the rest of your life. These foods can make you feel healthy, young, strong, and energetic. These foods stop the aging process, give you clarity in your mind, brain, and spirit. These foods boost your memory, eliminate most old-age diseases, and reverse the aging process by helping new cell growth all over your body and your entire system or your biological timer. Take my word, you will feel great and fantastic, confident, fit, and young.

Some old people who sometimes didn't pay attention to what they eat think that they missed the boat and it's probably too late or they are too old to start over or to attempt the reversal process. I say no! This is wrong for them to think like that; this is not true! To me, no matter how old you are, if you are still alive and even not too well, it's possible that you can ameliorate, cut back, slow down the progression of the aging process. All you have to do is add some of these good foods to your diet and decrease or eliminate some of the bad foods or not too good from your diet. Finally we are going to start with these good foods.

CRUCIFEROUS VEGETABLES

There is a group of vegetables called cruciferous, which are cabbage, cauliflower, broccoli, kale, turnips, brussels sprouts, radishes, and watercress. These vegetables flush toxin from your body, preventing these poisons from aging you before your natural and chronological age. These vegetables clean your system and throw out the poisons. These vegetables can restore your immune system to the same strength and fighting form that it had when you were young. These vegetables activate the sleeping genes and enzymes in your immune cells that can fight the harmful effects of dangerous molecules called free radicals, which can damage your body cells and tissue. These vegetables prevent wrinkles, provide a good skin turgor or elasticity, prevent and protect us from getting other diseases that come with old age. Remember at the beginning of the chapter about what makes people grow old. We will talk about the diseases and prevention of them in another chapter alphabetically.

WHOLE GRAIN

These are pasta, breads, cereals, waffles, pancakes, muffins made with barley, oatmeal, bran, and rice.

These foods are full of complex carbohydrates that are the building blocks of our body, vitamin B, and fiber that are converted to energy to boot. Thereby they can prevent low energy, one of the symptoms of aging. This energy is not the once-in-a-while or temporary kind. It's a constant supply throughout the day, weeks, months, and years. And this type of energy is provided without detrimental effects to your blood sugar levels, which is another problem as we get older. Therefore, eat four to five servings of whole grain a day of the products above. Remember that servings are measured in cups, half cups, a slice of bread, a small or medium size of pancake, waffle, and muffin. The above can be used in any meal and snack for the day and night.

NUTS, ALMONDS, SEEDS

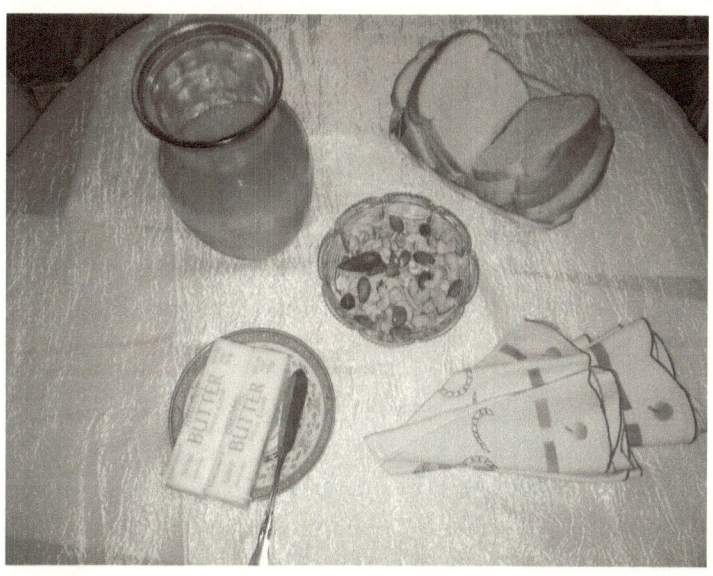

Nuts, almonds to be exact, contain substances called neurotransmitters that carry messages from cell to cell in the brain which makes your memory sharp and keen. Although nuts and almonds don't have all the neurotransmitters, they have the most powerful ones like dopamine that help your memory and make you feel happy. Your brain can make dopamine from a substance called phenylalanine that can be found in many other foods, which we will talk about later. Walnuts contain omega -3 fatty acids that nourishes a protective fat sheath in the brain called myelin. Brazil nuts boost your

immune system, which makes you healthy, help you fight infections, diseases, and molecules called free radicals that cause aging rapidly. Therefore, fight aging and stay young for many more years to come by eating a handful of brazil nuts and other nuts mixed together daily. Pumpkin seeds and flaxseeds contain the same substances that can make you feel and look young too.

Sunflower Seeds

Sunflower seeds contain vitamin E that protects the skin from damage caused by the sun and other toxins and pollutants in our environment. Vitamin E increases our production of collagen, a substance that keeps the skin soft, smooth, clear, clean, and radiant. Vitamin E also keeps our bones strong, our joints and tendons in solid and good working condition.

BLUEBERRIES

Blueberries contain powerful antioxidants called flavonoids, which protect all our body's cells from damage that causes premature aging. Therefore, eat blueberries and all food products made with blueberries, such as blueberry muffins, waffles, jelly, fruit juice, cereals, blueberry pie, and granola bars. Eat a handful of blueberries daily at any time of the day as a snack. Put some blueberry jelly with peanut butter in two slices of whole-grain bread to make a sandwich of complete plant protein. Two high proteins combined turn to a complete protein meal. We need protein but are afraid of saturated fat from animal protein. So our best choice is plant protein. Protein nourishes our cells that die by the thousands every minute. Therefore, we need to replace them with plant protein and less animal protein every minute also. If not, we get old rapidly, even more than our chronological age. We need to eat protein at least every twenty-four hours or less divided by two to three meals or times a day. We can find protein in whole grain, some vegetables, nuts, soy milk and tofu, and all animal products.

CARROTS

Carrots are rich in vitamin B, beta-carotene, which is good for our eyes, hair, and skin that the color would never be a pale shade when you eat *this vegetable. Eating carrots gives your skin a bright peachy, rosy, and orange lustrous hue like a natural makeup. Carrots protect your lungs from damage by tobacco smoke whether you smoke or not (which you shouldn't) or whether you inhale secondhand—or the newest, third hand—smoking and environmental pollutants. Eating carrots can make it easier for you to breathe and keep your body's cells in tiptop shape with oxygen that preserves youth. You can forget about COPD, asthma, cataract, alopecia, or baldness. With carrots, your pulse (through ox-meter, a medical instrument that measures the oxygen level in our blood) will always be 95 percent to 100 percent most of the time. Your eyes can be twenty-twenty with or without glasses and reverse your vision as when you were young. You will be able to read without glasses outside or with bright light inside except maybe for very fine prints in a dark room.*

Forget about baldness. Your hair will not fall from your head anymore.

And you will not need to wear wigs, toupees, hairpiece, and weaves. Your hair will grow a head full of lively, healthy, and strong new growth, which you can add a temporary rinse of your choice or leave as is to make you look ten to thirty years younger than your biological and chronological age.

AVOCADOS

Avocados, like carrots, can do the same for your hair, eyes, and skin because of the vitamin E that they contain. Avocados control your blood pressure, which is usually a big problem in old people. Eating avocados can keep your blood pressure at a level that can make your system look like and feel like a child or the most a twenty-year-old person with a 110/70 to a maximum of 120/80, the perfect blood pressure. Avocados, besides fighting wrinkles, blindness, blood pressure, erase hot flashes and other bad consequences of menopause, containing good fat that don't make you gain weight. You will be going through menopause unnoticed. Hot flashes, night sweats, and nasty mood swings will be banished for you.

GARLIC

Garlic not only keep you young, but can also save your life. Eating garlic raw in salad or cooked in meals in slices, powder, and oil can prevent you from having hearth diseases or cardiovascular problems that can kill you or leave you crippled and disabled. Garlic can reduce the fatty (LDL) cholesterol level and increase elasticity of your blood vessel walls, thereby permitting the blood to flow more efficiently through your arteries. Garlic can prevent you from having elevated or abnormal blood pressure. And if you already have high blood pressure or hypertension, garlic will regulate and decrease it. At your next visit to your doctor, he or she will be surprised, complimenting you and decreasing the amount of your drug. If you are lucky enough, you might not be on drugs anymore. There are other foods and herbs that are good for the same conditions that we will come to in other chapters in this book.

GINGER

Ginger is my number one spice and miracle remedy. You can't be young, feel young, and look young if you look puffy, bloated, have swelling, indigestion, and can't absorb the vitamins, minerals, and nutrients from your foods. But by drinking ginger tea at least twice a week and using fresh ginger root in some of your meals, dishes, snacks, and as candy or in trail mix daily or at least four to five times a week, you can be sure that your digestive system is in excellent condition to keep you young, alert, and energetic. Don't forget that ginger is the most powerful natural remedy in the proper assimilation of vitamins, minerals, and nutrients that your body needs.

WATERMELON

Watermelon is full of compounds that fight free radicals and vitamins A, B, C, E. It contains some mineral too, such as selenium, zinc, and fatty acids, quercetin, linolenic acid, and others that can fight aging by keeping your skin wrinkle free, nice, hydrated, and elastic. Watermelon is good for your eyes, hair, and promotes some sexual hormones that increase male and female libido.

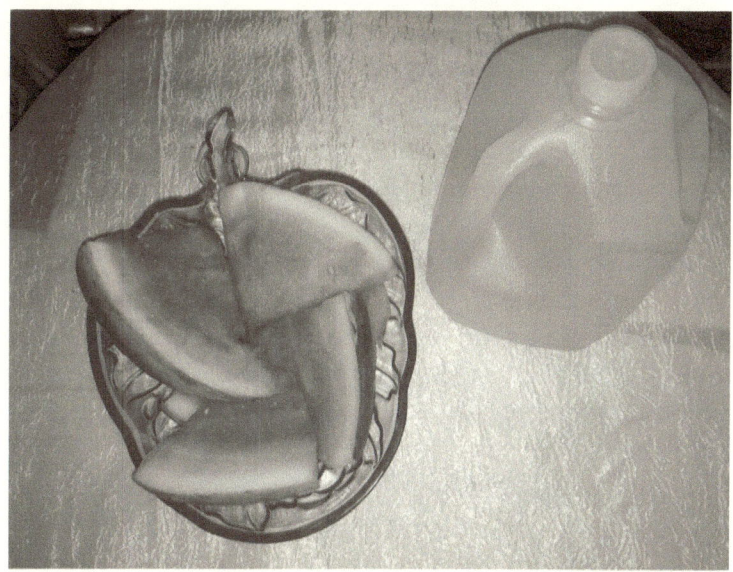

APPLE

To quote the old 1965 commercial, "New Kellogg's Apple Jacks, a bowl a day keeps the bullies away." I think that an apple a day keeps the doctors, the nurses, the CNA (certified nursing assistants), nursing homes, assisted-living homes, and home attendants away for a long time for some people. Apple is the first fruit in man's history as per the Bible and other religious history and scriptures. Apple, besides keeping you young, is good for preventing and alleviating many other diseases and conditions. We will talk about these conditions when we get to conditions alphabetically. For now, for keeping people young, apple is good for fighting cholesterol that produce plaques in your arteries and preventing cardiovascular diseases that make people age and die prematurely. Apple helps fight and prevent osteoporosis, which affects especially pre and postmenopausal women and makes them look and feel old and weak before their chronological age and time. Women can say good-bye to this type of suffering. Surprisingly, the apple doesn't have that many vitamins besides vitamin C. But apples contain enzymes, minerals, and fibers that make it the richest fruit in this category. Apple is good for almost every conditions and diseases, any age at any time of the day in any meal and any dish you want to prepare.

Apples contain high levels of quercetin, a powerful antioxidant that protect against memory loss, a major part of aging. Although some quercetin are in the flesh, the most of it is found in the apple's skin. Apples have enough antioxidants to raise the levels of acetylcholine, a neurotransmitter that's essential to memory and tends to decline with age.

Apples have many ways to be eaten. If you can't eat the whole fruit, you sure can eat a variety of apple preparations such as applesauce, apple pie, apple cake, apple juice, apple cider, apple vinegar, apple chips in your salad and condiment, apple drink, apple in your cereal, apple candy, apple fruit salad, apple trail mix, dry apple, jelly apple, apple butter, and many other ways that I can't name. Also, apples have the most brand names and types than any other fruits. Almost every day I go to the supermarkets, I noticed many different types and names and brands added to the apple family.

CONCLUSION OF FIGHTING AGING

To close this chapter, I would like to remind you that we all need to age healthily and gracefully since we are definitely getting old one day. As we grow older, our body composition changes, our muscles mass decreases because sometimes we don't use them that much. Meanwhile, our fatty tissues and flabby, loose skin increase. Since our metabolism slows down, we need to consume less fat and calories. Therefore, we need to decrease our calorie intake by 10 percent to 15 percent every decade after age forty. Some scientists say after fifty years old two decades ago. According to my research, observation, experience, and the new obesity epidemic, I say not just 10 percent after fifty years old, but 10 to 15 percent after forty years old and even more at fifty years old. Otherwise, it will be too late to start the fight against aging.

What you have to do is consume 10 percent less of the calories you used to in your thirtieth birthday, 15 percent calories in your fiftieth birthday, and up to eighty and over an additional 10 percent or 5 percent according to what you weigh. And especially if you don't exercise and are not too active. Since it's never too late to exercise, start doing strength exercise such as pulling, pushing, and weight lifting. Walk as much as you can to prevent and correct aging too fast and be unhealthy. Because if you don't do the above, you will be risking weight gain, obesity, heart diseases, diabetes type 2, osteoarthritis, and other diseases worse than looking and feeling old.

Since the body's ability to absorb nutrients decreases, older people need to eat foods with calcium, vitamin D, vitamin B12, other B vitamins, and E, zinc, potassium, and food rich in fiber to prevent gastrointestinal problems. Some of these problems are constipation, acid reflux, indigestion, gas, and mal absorption.

Foods to eat to prevent these problems and why are from all five groups in the pyramid.

Have four to five servings a day of this group.

Start with the largest group in the food pyramid, which are simple carbohydrates or starch and complex carbohydrates, such as whole-grain breads, cereals, waffles, pancakes, brown rice, and any colored rice except white, petit mil or millet, barley, oats and other whole grains and wheat, and bran. Eat dried beans of all colors, peas, lentils, legumes, potatoes, wheat pastas, and some other starchy foods sparingly for serotonin, thiamine, riboflavin, niacin, folate, B6, other B vitamins and complete protein meals when combined with beans and legumes.

Have five to six servings of fresh vegetables and fruits, such as the following:

Dark green leafy vegetables like spinach, kale, collard greens, mustard green, lettuce, broccoli, cabbage, carrots, squash, green beans, and all other vegetables.

Fruits: citrus fruits, berries, bananas, plums, prunes, pineapples, tomatoes, avocados for vitamins C, A, beta-carotene, riboflavin, folic acid, minerals, water, and fibers.

Protein Foods

Have two servings of lean beef, lamb, goat, chicken, turkey, other poultry, seafood, fish, eggs, or plant protein combined with grain to make a complete protein meal. You can benefit from these foods vitamins E, B6, B12, zinc, and some other minerals.

Dairy Products

Have two to three servings of fat-free or low-fat milk, cheese, yogurt, other milk products such as soy and lactose-reduced milk, cheese, and yogurt depending on your need. From these products, you can benefit from protein, calcium, vitamins A and D that old people need for preventing bone loss and other problems more than younger people. Older people need dairy products for preventing hair and teeth loss also.

RECOMMENDATION

It's a fact that we all are going to be old whether we like it or not, if we live that long. But we don't have to look old, feel old, act old, and lose our mind. Laughter adds to our vitality, and it takes more muscles to frown than to smile. The same way we exercise our muscles, joints, and ligaments physically, we should exercise our brain mentally, our emotions sanely, and our soul spiritually. The same way we want our body to be in shape and fit, we need our emotions to be adequate, our mind to be keen, and our brain to be functioning to the highest level also. Guess what? Our brain doesn't count the years of our biological and chronological timer or clock. We can be old by years and not by look or action. Just like toddlers play with other toddlers and also with grandpa, grandma, or with great-grandpa and great-grandma without prejudice or discrimination.

Therefore, I encourage people to follow some simple but important steps:

1. *Be active socially, mentally, emotionally, spiritually, and physically. Exercise your brain even more than your body. Keep abreast, sharp, and up-to-date. Never pass a day without reading something; writing something; playing some games; listening to some news or music; watching the news, a documentary, game show, educative program; and learning something new or old even from a child.*
2. *Go back to school, any school, to learn new things or to review old ones. Better yet if possible, do like some people—never stop at all. If needed, take a time-out or rest whatever you want to call it, but don't stay too long to lose track. If you can't go nonstop, take a semester or two from going physically to the school building; just take credits by correspondence or online on your computer. If you*

don't have a computer, go to the library to learn how to use one for schoolwork, checking your e-mail, have a Web site, or play a game. Young children are very good in these new technology and would be happy to play games with and teach older people. If you have a computer at home and know how to use it, do whatever you know how on it as much as possible and as often as you can. Even if it's a half hour to two hours every other day, it's better than nothing at all.

3. *Have a cell phone and use it to send and receive text messages, voice messages, voice mail; send your pictures to your loved ones to let them know that you are alive and well and missing them. When you are around them, use your camera and make videos of the time that you are together, and once in a while, watch the videos that can keep you company when you are alone. If you can't see, having someone record the voices and laughter of loved ones and friends to listen to will help you cope with loneliness and difficult times.*

4. *If you can read with or without glasses, read some good articles from your favorite magazines, do puzzles, crosswords, word finding, Illusion Confusion, brain teasers, table games with other people, millionaires, Jeopardy, and Wheel of Fortune. And shout the answers out from the top of your lungs. Play table games, board games, charade once or twice a month at least.*

5. *Learn to play a musical instrument, a foreign language from books, a school, and a native from that country where the language originated so you can also practice it verbally at least twice a week. Read the Bible or whatever book pertains to your faith, meditate, and pray.*

6. *Have a hobby, such as drawing, painting, gardening, flower work or arrangement, sewing, photographing, and writing a journal, short story, a dream book, a food journal, or diary. Do brisk walks or strolls, pacing, dancing, yoga, strength exercise, swimming for thirty minutes to one hour at least four to seven days a week depending on your ability and how you feel. You know yourself more than anyone else. You are the boss of your body and your brain. You tell your body and your brain what to do. Just be fair and treat them right. And never push yourself too hard, never abuse or take advantage of your body and your brain because you will regret it later on.*

7. *Have a good support system of family, friends, coworkers and neighbors. Be part of a social network of all ages, races, nationality, work of life, professions, and never discriminate. Because when you do, you give your brain the wrong signal. And please never stay at all times with people of your age only with the same problems, the same disability, the same race, the same society, and the same everything. You will be missing too much knowledge, fun, and adaptation. Also, if you do that, you will close the learning process, you will leave no room for growth, you will definitely be plateau, will stay stagnant, and limit yourself to the same level the most part of your life.*

8. *Of course, I know you need a routine. We all do. But a variety in doing certain things is the best to stay young, prevent aging, fight age deterioration, and delay the process. The routine comes in some needs such as sleep time at night or day, which the hours are seven to eight hours at night time and better, if possible, at the same time and place to go to bed, which is the best. Since seven to eight hours seem to be the magic number for adults and older people to sleep, we have to prepare ourselves for that to happen. Because if we sleep for nine, ten, to eleven hours or too many hours per night and day either straight or with interruption, we can harm ourselves the same way as too little sleep, such as from one to even six hours a night or day. Up to seven or seven and a half hours once in a while is not too bad. Therefore we all need a sleeping goal.*

To help achieve the sleeping goal, do the following:

1. *Start your preparation at the same time, give yourself some time ahead before you become sleepy. Take a bath, a shower or a washcloth in a washbasin and wash yourself, or do nothing, whatever is good for you. Brush your teeth or rinse your mouth or whatever goes with you. Get your sleeping gear made of cotton, silk, or nylon according to the season. It can be pajamas, gown, or T-shirt, it doesn't matter. But it shouldn't be too tight and have no strings to strangle you or block your circulation while sleeping. Make the room temperature comfortable for you, meaning from seven to seventy-two degrees Fahrenheit, which is just cool. But if you like it a little warmer, it's fine too. Except that the room shouldn't be too cold or too hot.*

2. *Some people like noise, such as music, which should be instrumental, with no lyrics to sing along. Just listen until you fall asleep. Reading should be good too. But only short stories, magazines, pamphlets, flyers, or poems. Because you need something short. Never read textbooks; big novels; romance; violent stories; war stories; sad, complicated documentaries; or learning materials; or brain teasers. You can use earplugs or listen to a steady noise maker such as in CDs or VHS and cassettes like rainwater on a rooftop, ocean waves, or a calm and slow wind in a forest.*

3. *Don't go to bed hungry. Eat a snack at least one hour before bedtime if you need to. Eat some foods with tryptophan, potassium, protein dairy, or plant protein such as a piece of a large banana or a small one; one half of a peanut butter sandwich with or without blueberry or grape jelly. Be careful of too much sugar, salty, and fatty foods. You can eat four ounces of cereal dry or with four ounces cup of milk. You can drink one eight-ounce cup of warm or cold milk. Eat a scoop of ice cream of any flavor except chocolate, coffee, or rum raisin or a piece of low-fat or fat-free cheese made of skimmed milk with 2 to 3 percent sodium at the most.*

4. *Do your own ritual, which can be meditation, imagery, or prayer of your own faith. Because whatever is in this book is good for everyone of any faith, religion, race, nationality. It's just to be healthy. And if you want to sleep a good seven and a half to eight hours nonstop, remember to go to the bathroom to urinate right before you hit the sack.*

5. *Last, remember not to do physical activities or brain activity up to three hours before going to bed to sleep. Do only deep breathing exercises to relax and relaxation exercises if you know how to fall asleep in a short time. If you don't know how to do relaxation exercises, refer to my other book* T.H.A.T.S., The Health Assistance to Some. *You can go to the Web site Mariethats.com or call (516) 835-1598 to buy the book.*

ALCOHOL, ALCOHOLISM, ALCOHOLIC

Alcohol

Alcohols are organic compounds formed from hydrocarbon by substituting one or more hydroxyl groups for a similar number of hydrogen atoms.

Ethyl alcohol is colorless, volatile, a flammable liquid of the formula C_2H_5OH. The molecular weight for it is 46.07, boiling point is 78.5 degrees Centigrade. Alcohol is in fermented or distilled liquors and is obtained in its pure form from fermentation and fractionation distillation.

Property and Use of Alcohol

We use alcohol to make tincture extracts, manufacturing of ether, ethylene, and industrial products, such as rubbing alcohol compound, antiseptic when in 70 percent solution. Alcohol stops growth of putrefactive bacteria and is used as preservative of biological specimens and in certain medicines. It's used in antifreeze products because of its low freezing point. Instruments can be sterilized when placed in a 70 percent solution of alcohol for thirty minutes. Alcohol is a depressant to the nervous system when drunk in large amounts. It can be used in IV solutions to stop premature labor.

ALCOHOLIC

This is a person who is affected with alcoholism.

Side Effects

Alcoholic psychosis is a severe mental disorder caused by drinking too much alcohol that can turn to a pathological intoxication, delirium tremens, Korsakoff's psychosis, and acute hallucinations.

ALCOHOLISM

Alcoholism is a chronic progressive and potentially fatal disease. It is characterized by tolerance and physical dependency or pathological organ changes or both. Below is a list of direct consequences for a person who drinks alcohol heavily:

1. Chronic and progressive means that the physical, emotional, social changes that develop are accumulative and the person keeps drinking more, continuously.
2. Tolerance means the brain adapts to high concentrations of alcohol.

3. The person has physical dependency and withdrawal symptoms that occur from decreasing or stopping from drinking alcohol suddenly.

4. The alcoholic can't consistently predict drinking occasions, circumstances, how long the person is going to drink, and how much he or she will drink and can drink.

5. Pathological organ changes can be found in almost any organ and system, especially in the brain, the liver, the pancreas, urinary tract, kidney, nervous system, peripheral nervous system, cardiopulmonary system, and gastrointestinal tract.

6. Drinking pattern is generally continuous but can be intermittent; sometimes the person stops for a period of time and starts again for apparently no reason.

7. Social, emotional, and behavioral symptoms and consequences of alcoholism result from the effects of alcohol on the function of the brain. The degree to which these symptoms and signs are considered deviant will depend upon the cultural norms of the society or group in which the person lives, works, or associates with.

8. Some physical signs and symptoms are motor instability or staggered gait, blurred or double vision, impaired reflex action, reduced mental function, increased pulse rate, decreased blood pressure, dilated pupils, flushing of skin, drowsiness or stupor, malnutrition, vitamin deficiency, alcoholic cirrhosis of the liver, gastritis, pancreatitis, neurological disorders such as tremulousness, hallucination, seizures, and delirium tremens.

ETIOLOGY

The etiology of alcoholism is unknown. All we know up to 2010 is that psychological, physiological, and sociological factors play an important part. Exhilaration factor is often the cause of intoxication in normal average people. Alcoholism is an illness and like any other disease or illness should be and can be treated. We also know that if left untreated, alcoholism can cause death.

MORE INFORMATION ABOUT ALCOHOL

Before we start with treatment and nutrition, we need to know some more information about alcohol, some good and some bad.

Drinking alcohol in moderation is not bad at all. In fact, a glass or two of an alcoholic beverage once in a while can raise your good cholesterol HDL level and cuts your risk of having a heart attack, improve your digestion, and put you in a good and happy mood.

Drawbacks

Alcohol drinking can interact with some medications and can increase the risk of some diseases such as cancer, stroke, heart disease, liver disease, kidney disease, dementia, and psychosis. People had been using alcohol a long time ago for different purposes, for example, to feel happy, subdue, as anesthetic, disinfectant, and tonic in a lot of medications. Most alcohols are made from potatoes, grains, honey, grapes, sugarcane, and most fruits. Unlike foods, alcohol can't be digested. A great percent of alcohol is absorbed in the bloodstream from the stomach, the small intestine, in about an hour after digestion. The rest of the alcohol in the body is eliminated through the kidneys, the lungs, and the skin. The liver breaks down or metabolizes alcohol. The time this takes depend on if the person drinks while eating, the person's sex, weight, body type, and tolerance level, which increases with how long the person has been drinking. Usually the liver takes three to four hours to metabolize an ounce of alcohol. The liver takes its time to process the alcohol drip by drip like a leaky faucet. Hard liquors, whiskey, and gin cause a faster impact on the body than wines and beers. And all kinds of alcohol is absorbed very fast if mixed with carbonated beverage like club soda or carbonated soft drinks. As soon as the alcohol in your bloodstream reaches the brain, it acts as a stimulant and produces euphoria. It makes you feel numb, sleepy, or unconscious. If people drink too much alcohol too fast, it can kill them.

What Some Researchers Say and Some Factors Pertaining to Alcoholism

Some researchers say that small amounts of wine, especially red wine, and drinking moderately can lower the fatty cholesterol (LDL) low density lipoprotein level because of a substance in red wine called bioflavonoids, an antioxidant.

Some factors pertaining to alcoholism are genetic predisposition, learned behavior, bad experiences in early childhood by using alcohol abuse as a coping mechanism. The process to become an alcoholic is different from person to person. Some people become alcoholic after the first drink or as they begin to drink. Others take a long drinking time to be addicted to alcohol.

Alcohol Effects on Nutrition

The alcoholics need all kinds of vitamins and nutrients from bottles because not only do they not take time to eat good foods, their digestion and absorption of nutrients from foods are also lousy. They have the poorest diets that cause bad digestion and metabolism of almost all nutrients. They lack of all enzymes, vitamins, and nutrients, especially thiamine, which can give them muscle cramps, wasting, nausea, vomiting, loss of appetite, nerve problems, depression, and psychosis. Very often, the alcoholics don't have enough folate, vitamin B6, riboflavin, selenium, vitamin A, which can cause blindness, vitamin D, which metabolizes calcium and other minerals that can cause bone loss, fractures, and diseases such as osteoporosis. The alcoholics can't digest fat, and function of the liver and pancreas is very poor. Because alcohol activates insulin production, glucose metabolism increases faster and results in low blood sugar or hypoglycemia. Some alcoholics are overweight or obese because alcohol contains a lot of calories.

TREATMENT

Stop drinking is a must. As soon as the alcoholic stops drinking, solution for the diet problems must be worked at and solved one by one. All deficiencies in nutrition must be corrected and converted with a good diet that can prevent the person from gaining weight. Other problems with pancreas and liver should be addressed. Fat and protein intake should be controlled to prevent damages to these organs. The best treatment for alcoholism is to stop drinking completely and continue to stay sober. Alcoholics need all the help they can get to achieve these goals from detoxification agencies or rehab facilities, different groups, organizations, family, and friends. The alcoholics need to stay away from people and places where alcohol is served and who is drinking it and where they can find drinks easily. Stay away from places where you can find alcoholic drinks easily and friends or anyone who drinks alcohol and can be tempted to drink it too.

Strategies

Get a habit such as gardening, painting, drawing, learning to play an instrument, singing, dancing, exercising, and learning a new language. Get a project with people in church or any faith where there is an assembly building around other people. Go to concerts, theaters where there are a lot of people. Don't be alone or not doing something with some other people. Keep yourself occupied. With or without people, watch funny movies, be with people who crack jokes, read funny magazines, and be in public places with other people and make new friends who don't drink. Destroy all drinking reminders, places, time, objects, and relationships with people who drink. Be a new you and never be sad, alone, or lonely. Be happy, joyful, and full of energy, which you didn't have for some time.

DIET

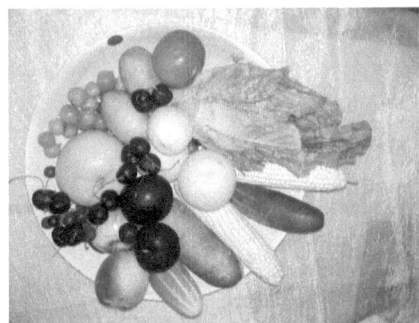 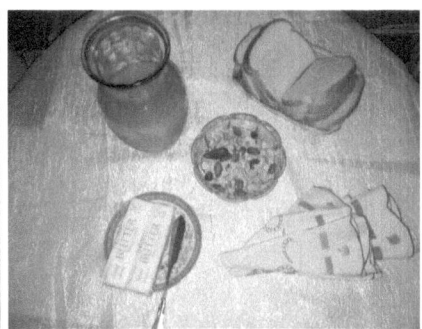

Eat food of all groups in moderation, whole grains, wheat, barley, oats, bread, and cereal and pasta made of grains, brown rice, beans of all colors, etc., with complex carbohydrates and fiber about four to five servings a day.

Eat fruits and vegetables of all kinds that you like, your vegetable steamed, boiled, or stir-fried but not fried. Get four to six servings of fruits and vegetables per day. Serving are one cup or one-half cup or a slice or a wedge of large fruits and small whole fruits two to three per day or raw vegetable salad one bowl per day. Drink fruit juices one or two glasses of 100 percent natural and no sugar added.

Eat only lean protein and plant protein such as fat-trimmed piece of steak the size of the palm of a child or four ounces. Eat chicken breast baked, four ounces or two drumsticks, three wings, one thigh, or whatever part you like, but no more than five ounces. Stew your meat with vegetables such as all-colored sweet peppers. Eat ground turkey meat or breast well cooked. Eat grilled seafood or fish mostly, such as salmon and others.

For dairy, drink only low-fat, fat-free, or skimmed milk. Eat fat-free or low-fat skimmed milk cheese, soy products, and yogurt moderately. Use salt or sodium and sugar moderately. Replace these two with mixed-blend spices with no salt, ginger, cinnamon, curry, garlic, onion, thyme, clove, black pepper, and hot pepper or hot sauce, and hot spicy mustard to revive your appetite and your taste buds, which were cooked and destroyed by long-term alcohol drinking.

SUPPORT SYSTEM

Go to group meetings like Alcoholics Anonymous for yourself and send your family members if you still have some to different-named groups that you can find online and in phone books.

Drink spring water or any good water you can have except the ones called sugar water and vitamin water by seven to eight eight-ounce cup or glass per day to hydrate you and flush the toxins from your body. Drink natural 100 percent fruit juices with no sugar added. Go to the gym, exercise, walk daily, climb stairs, sleep seven to eight hours a day. Play table games with family or in organizations; go to organized trips, theaters, and movies with nonalcoholic people.

For more information about good foods, how to cook your foods, how to protect your food and make a well-balanced meal, how to exercise, and a lot more of exercises and practice, go to Mariethats.com to obtain the previous book T.H.A.T.S., The Health Assistance to Some.

ALKALOSIS

This is a condition due to excessive alkalinity of body fluids due to accumulation of alkali or reduction of acids. It's the complete reverse of acidosis. Alkalosis has to do with blood pH balance, acid base balance, body fluids, and electrolyte balance. There are two types of alkalosis: metabolic alkalosis and respiratory alkalosis.

Metabolic Alkalosis

The alkalosis in which the pH balance of body fluids is increased and serum carbon dioxide content is greater than seventy volumes percent of (30 mEq/L) 30 milli equivalent per liter. Commonly, it's a result of loss of acid from excessive vomiting, loss of potassium, or ingestion of excessive amounts of sodium bicarbonate. Symptoms are apathy, irritability, delirium, dehydration, and sometimes tetanus.

Treatment or prevention: To replenish your potassium level, eat or drink juices and shakes from foods rich in potassium, such as bananas, potatoes, cantaloupes, and others. For the acid, drink citrus fruit juices, eat tomatoes, pineapples, and most fruits that contain a lot of vitamin C. Drink seven to eight eight-ounce cups of spring water to prevent dehydration, rest and decrease stress by using meditation, decreasing stimuli by staying in a quiet, dark, and comfortable room without disturbance to decrease irritability.

Respiratory Alkalosis

Respiratory alkalosis is when the pH body fluids are increased but the serum carbon dioxide content is less than 21 mEq/L (21 milli equivalent per liter). This condition is caused by hyperventilation; salicylate poisoning, lesion of the central nervous system, or decreased oxygen content of the air. Symptoms are lightheadedness, fainting, and tetanus.

Treatment

Discontinue use of salicylate; there is poisoning usually in some medications. Inhalation of expired CO_2 collected by breathing into a paper bag (in case of neurosis); correction or alleviation of the central nervous system disorder or lesion. Sometimes hyperventilation occurs or hyperpnea in forced respiration, increased inspiration and expiration of air as a result of increase in rate or depth of respiration, or both inspiration and expiration. Results in carbon dioxide depletion (acapnia) with accompanying symptoms are as *follows: fall in blood pressure, vasoconstriction, syncope, which is usually accompanied of marked anxiety.*

Immediate Treatment

Have the person breathe into a paper bag until the CO_2 content of the blood has the opportunity to return to normal. Just as effective is to close one nostril and be certain the person breathes with his or her mouth closed. In both cases, this person needs to be reassured and calmed.

And now to prevent these situations or conditions before they happen or after, not to reappear, these are what you are going to do or not to do:

1. *Know about acid/alkali imbalance. Acidity and alkalinity are measured according to the pH balance. PH for water is 7.0 neutral. The ideal human pH is between 6.0 and 6.8. Below 6.3 for body pH is acidic. Above pH 6.8 is alkaline.*
2. *Acid and alkaline self-test. This test determines whether your body fluids are too acidic or too alkaline. You can purchase litmus paper at most drugstores without prescription and apply saliva or urine to the paper. The paper will change color to indicate if your system is overly acidic or alkaline. Red litmus paper turns blue in an alkaline medium. Blue litmus paper turns red in an acidic medium. Always perform the test either before eating or after at least one hour after eating. If your test indicates that your body is too acidic, consult the recommendation to follow under "Acidosis," which we already covered in the previous chapter.*
3. *Know foods that are alkaline and foods that are acidic and balance them. Always read food labels to know their content of salt, sodium, and acid.*
4. *The best anyone can do is to eat a large variety of foods with a limited portion. Too much of any type of foods is bad. Always match your intake with each other to balance it. When preparing your meals, take a look at both groups, the acidic and the alkaline group, and pick some foods in both. Know that dairy products and soft drinks with carbonated gas are alkaline. Therefore, compose your daily diet intake with some alkaline and some acidic foods.*

List of Alkaline-Forming Foods

Corn
Avocado
Dates
Fresh coconut
Most fresh fruits
Most fresh vegetables
Onions
Potatoes
Rutabagas
Honey
Horseradish
Maple syrup
Molasses
Raisins
Soy products
Sprouts
Plums
Watercress

Some raw vegetables and some citrus fruits can do both at the same time, acidify and alkalinize in the system.

Low-Level Alkaline-Forming Foods:

Almonds
Brazil nuts
Chestnuts
Lima beans
Petit mil or millet
Soured dairy products

Do not make a complete daily-intake meals with the following foods alone:

Milk
Cheese
Mashed potatoes

Yogurt
Cottage cheese
White bread
Peanut butter
Avocado
Coconut juice
Mushroom
Soy products as protein to replace meat
Honey
Raisin
Watercress

WHY? This is a good question! Because if you do, you will have complete alkaline meals for the entire day, which can be dangerous. Remember that knowledge is power. Therefore, you need to go to the acidic foods chart or list and cook meat, poultry, fish, or plant protein, dry beans, brown rice, cabbage, bell pepper of all colors, kale, broccoli, eggs, lentils, chickpeas, asparagus, buckwheat, catsup, cranberries, mustard, noodles, pasta, oatmeal, olives, plums, prunes, sauerkraut, sugar, sugar-added food, tea drinks, coffee, fruit juices, lemonade, wine or alcoholic beverages moderately and sparingly, eat tomato, romaine lettuce, add vinegar or vinaigrette to your salad as you wish. The bottom line is if you do not know about acid and alkaline from the first book T.H.A.T.S., *go to the food list in this book and mix your foods with each other from the five groups in the food pyramid. Make a food menu for every day of the week for your own cooking or to eat out. It is the only way to be on the safe side of healthy nutrition and prevent acidosis and alkalosis among other diseases and conditions. Check for recipes at the end of this book or refer to the previous book* T.H.A.T.S., The Health Assistance to Some.

RECOMMENDATIONS

Use a diet that consists of 80 percent grains, whole ones including beans, breads, brown rice, crackers, lentils, pastas, nuts, whole-grain cereals. Use the other 20 percent of the diet by including fresh fruits, vegetables, fish, chicken, turkey, eggs, natural reduced-fat cheese, milk, non-trans fat margarine and oils. Do not use too much antacids or mineral supplements. Avoid salt and sodium, or use it sparingly or what is naturally in the foods.

Cut back on vitamins from a bottle and minerals too. Know that your foods, if well protected by the food protection program from T.H.A.T.S. program based on the U.S. Health Department, if your meals are made of a large variety of natural, organic, fresh-produces, fat-free, or reduced-fat dairy, meat, and poultry, you will be fine and healthy. Because you will find all the vitamins and minerals that your body needs just from the foods you eat and not necessarily from bottles of pills.

EXERCISE

Do not do prolonged deep-breathing exercises. Do not hyperventilate, decrease stress, don't be too anxious, relax and calm down more often. Listen to soft music, practice yoga; if you feel out of breath while exercising, stop and catch your breath, get out if inside or open the doors or windows, and put your head out and breathe the fresh air with oxygen. If you are inside and can't get out but feel anxious or stressed out, breathe in a paper bag because the above are symptoms of alkalosis.

Stop smoking tobacco or cigarettes. Stop drinking alcoholic beverages permanently or until the condition you are having stops. And don't forget to stop all drugs, see your doctor, and test your alkaline and acid with the litmus paper daily.

Living Condition

If you live in a crowded and polluted city, go to the suburbs, in the woods, backyard, or waterside or beach or pool and lakes and ocean side on your days off or vacation time to breathe cleaner, fresher air full of oxygen to enrich your red blood cells and fight alkalosis. Meditate to relieve anxiety. Do imagery or hypnosis, slow down your activities of daily living, and have some fun to decrease stress. Be happy with what you have, laugh at something funny, and be wise and make what you have to do for you or benefit you from a bad situation and turn it around to a good situation. Be positive, optimistic, and hopeful and say to yourself it could have been worse and the grass is not really always greener on the other side of the fence.

ALLERGY

Allergy is an acquired hypersensitivity to certain substances called allergens that don't normally cause a reaction. While it's essentially an antibody-antigen reaction, in some cases, the antibody can't be demonstrated. The reaction is due to the release of histamine or histamine-like substances from injured cells. It can be a genetic predisposition to acquire a particular allergy. The amount or number of exposure necessary to produce enough antibodies to cause an allergy varies. An allergy may occur the second time a person is exposed to a particular allergen or may not occur until years later, when repeated exposures have produced sufficient antibodies. Manifestations most commonly involve the respiratory tract or the skin.

Allergic Reactions and Symptoms

Some allergic reactions are eczema; allergic rhinitis (running nose) or coryza; hay fever; bronchial asthma; urticaria; hives; eosinophilia; nasal congestion; tearing; sneezing; wheezing; coughing; itching rash; eruptions; nausea; vomiting; swelling in the mouth, throat, skin, and mucous membrane; and anaphylactic shock.

Allergen

Allergen is any substance that causes manifestation of allergy. It may not be a protein or an antigen. Some common allergens are inhalants, dusts, pollen, fungi, smoke, perfumes, odors of plastics, fragrances, deodorants, some medications like antibiotics, aspirin, serums, narcotics, antidepressant, contraceptives, vitamins, nutrients. Other allergens are infectious agents, bacteria, viruses, fungus, animal parasites, contactants, chemical agents, detergents, soaps, bleach, cosmetics, heat, cold, light, pressure, radiation, clothes, leather, nylon, silk, hair, fur, feathers, wool, chemicals, insect bites, some toothpastes, mouthwash, rubber gloves, condoms, and even stress can cause an allergic reaction to a person. Some people can be allergic to some sounds, odors, or smells. People can be allergic to common pets: dogs, cats, rodents, birds, fish, or lizards. People can be allergic to plants, fresh flowers, fresh-cut grass, crabgrass, weeds, and trees.

Foods That Cause Allergic Reactions

Some specific foods causing allergic reactions are eggs, chocolate, milk, wheat, tomatoes, citrus fruits, oatmeal, potatoes, nuts, peanuts, corn, rice, fish, shellfish, seafood, lamb meat, honey, artificial sweeteners, some syrups, some spices and vegetables, some water bottles if purified with charcoal or iodine, some ingredients in processed foods, carbonated soft drinks, dye, and some artificial flavors.

GOOD ADVICE

Make sure you read labels every time you shop for any product and not just the newly used ones. Because you might be using the same products for many years and find out that something else is added to them. For instance, you may be allergic to milk, eggs, and the sunlight. But what are these things have in common? The answer is vitamin D. Some people are allergic to vitamin D and don't even know. Fortunately, others find out by accident or repeated symptoms when exposed to sunlight and think that they are allergic to sunlight. In reality, these people are probably allergic to vitamin D in the sun and in some foods.

Interview

When I ask these people with symptoms to sunlight, what about eating cheese, eggs, yogurt and drinking milk? Some answer, "Come to think of it, I don't react too well with these foods either. I don't particularly like them." "Why?" "Because after I eat or drink them, I feel uncomfortable. I feel my throat getting sore, tied, or closing, my eyes watery and my skin itchy. But it stops after some time all by itself."

Some people know for sure that they are allergic to the sun and can't eat some dairy products. At least, I know ten individuals I had been following for years who have the same reactions to sunlight exposure and eating and drinking some dairy products. These are one adult and nine children. Let's start with the adult.

Adult Case Number 1

Mr. Warren in his fifties is an adult male, of the black race from Barbados. When this gentleman asked me what to do to keep in shape and not feel too tired so often, I said to walk daily for good health. He answered, "It's hard for me to walk because I work from 3:00 PM to 11:00 PM." I said to him, "Why can't you walk before work time?" He said, "No, because since I was a child, I can't stay outside under the sunlight. I get blisters and a burning sensation even if I wear pants, long-sleeved shirts, and hat. I have these blisters on my hands and have to wear gloves in the heat. So I usually walk at night or very early in the morning before sunrise."

Child Number 1

The first child I noticed with a sunlight problem is a neighbor's two-year-old boy named Erick. I was on my way to work by walk and left many hours ahead of time. While passing by a woman holding on to a child one block down, I heard a loud screaming, a shrill noise, and noticed the child pulling away from the mother who was holding on to him. This child was practically white from a German male and an African American woman who had met him while on vacation in Germany. As a result, this child was conceived. Fortunately for the child, the woman had high blood pressure and could not have an abortion. She had a husband and three other children with him. The girls were brown skinned. Therefore, this last child, a boy, needed a shade darker from the sunlight in order to pass as the couple's only son.

When I looked at the child closely, I noticed that his body was all blistery and burned from the sunlight. The poor child was in pain. I took him inside the house, gave him a cool bath, dried him up with a soft cloth, applied baby powder on his body, placed him in a crib with a cold bottle of apple juice, and waited until he finished drinking and fell asleep. The mother asked me if I could help her with other housework also for pay. I said yes but only temporary and I didn't want her money. That day, I cleaned the kitchen, washed dishes, straightened up the countertop, placed toys and dirty clothes in the proper place, and mopped the floors, prepared meals for the sick child and the other children in school. I made farina for Erick and asked the woman for fresh milk. Instead, she gave me a box of formula from the refrigerator and told me that the child was allergic to dairy products. I said to myself, "Ah-ah, he is allergic to the sun also, therefore he must be allergic to vitamin D."

I took Erick under my wing and followed him until adulthood. Eventually, the mother and the mother's husband got a divorce. The German gentleman came to the USA with his wife and daughter and lived for some time incognito in a few blocks away from Erick and his mother. One day, the child requested that I call his father for him. I did, but the father wasn't home and his wife answered the phone. Erick grabbed the phone from me and said, "Hi, Daddy." The lady said, "He doesn't have a son. He only has one child, a daughter who is right here with me." By the time I got the phone from Erick, the woman screamed and passed out. A few months later, this German man came to my house and told me that his wife had divorced him because of that phone call I made for Erick. I feel sorry for his wife and daughter, but happy for Erick who finally got both parents living with him and three half sisters visiting him.

I continued until the present to investigate and research on my own and find out many people, adults and children, who are afflicted with this type of allergy. But I can only name a few cases and move on. I have four more children in addition to Erick to make five cases and one more adult female, in addition to the gentleman from the island.

Child Number 2: Girl Named Sacha

A two-year-old African American girl used to bite, scratch, kick, and scream if anyone tried to pick her up to take her to the park to play or walk under the sunlight. Even with clothes and a large brimmed hat covering her entire body and face, it didn't make any difference to her. One day at the daycare that she attended, one of the teachers called Sacha's mother who came and said, "Oh, she is always like that, she doesn't like the sunlight and is afraid of it because it burns her and causes blisters on her exposed body parts."

Child Number 3: Bobby

A four-year-old white boy who likes to swim in the pool for hours was shivering from the cold water and had his lips turned blue but wouldn't sit outside to warm up. When I questioned the mother, she said, "Oh, Bobby is

*always like that, doesn't like the sunlight, gets burned, turns red and blistery."
"What about dairy products, can he consume them?" I asked. "Oh no, he can't drink cow's milk, eat cheese or ice cream. They make him itchy all over." As a teen, I continued to follow Bobby, and one day I saw the mother sitting in front of her house real late at night. I asked, "Why are you outside so late?" She said, "I am waiting for Bobby to come back from his walk. He can only walk late at night because of the sunlight. He is still afraid of it."*

Child Number 4

Lizette Spanish, a six-year-old girl, came to an after-school program, crying, turning red and scratching her skin out from her arms, hands, legs, and face. When asked, her older sister named Christine said, "Oh, she doesn't like the sun, and we missed the bus today we had to walk here. She doesn't drink cow's milk or eat cheese. She drinks soy milk."

Child Number 5

Channel, a very smart three-year-old little African American girl, wouldn't go outside without her large brimmed cloth hat, long pants, and long-sleeved shirt. She doesn't cry, but make sure to sit under the shade while outside in the park playing. She usually sits close to the teachers and buried her face on their shoulders or laps.

All these boys and girls from different races and nationalities have the same common behaviors. The point that I am trying to make is this: people should be careful about putting a single product or vitamin in every food. Because most of the time, people who are allergic to the sun are also allergic to dairy products with vitamin D added to them. It's not that bad if these people use the dairy products with the natural vitamin D originally in the products. Some people don't get sick from this kind of vitamin D. But when the vitamin D is from a bottle or added to the food products, it can be devastating.

Adult Case Number 2

Another problem arises when people continue to eat the same foods every day or too much. They start to have some bad reactions to the same foods they have been eating for years. Their body has enough of the same foods and reacts to them. What people in that case must do is to stop eating these foods for a while and change them for other new foods. Then after some time, go back to them again. But this time, don't eat them every day. Eat them one day of the week and wait until day five of the same week, leaving four days in between. By doing this trick, you can prevent, decrease, and cure symptoms that can be hard to diagnose or detect except by a good investigator, diary keeper, and labels reader. I discovered this case in an adult woman, my friend, a doctor. She has been eating probiotic yogurt every day and many times a day for quite some time. She developed acidity, gas, stomach ulcer, abdominal cramp, and other stomach problems. When I talked to her recently, she said to me, "I think that I am allergic to sour foods." I said to her, "You are not, you just ate them too much and too often. And anything you eat too much good or bad can harm you. What you have to do is to slow down with this type of foods for a while and go back to them moderately and not as often as before. Give your system a break from these foods. Even if they are good foods, you can get sick from eating them too much and too often."

TREATMENT

Some treatments are skin test at a doctor's clinic to make sure of substances that a person is allergic to. Have a food diary to record what you eat daily and what new foods or new products, objects, places, people introduced to your environment and diet. Observe for anything newly introduced to your life in order to eliminate the allergens. Do the food diary for at least three weeks to find out what causes an allergic reaction when you eat food. Next, avoid all possible known allergens. For the allergens that can't be avoided, their effects can be lessened or decreased with medications like antihistamines, epinephrine, or corticosteroids. There is a process called desensitization that is still not clear. Remember that the best way to protect yourself is prevention and elimination of allergens by observing, analyzing, taking notes in your diary. When you have a reaction to something unknown, stay away from it. And don't eat something known by you that you like if you are allergic to it because allergic reactions progress or decrease.

Recommendation

Although a lot of foods are good for anyone, the same foods can also be some allergens for the same person. But what I can recommend for everyone is to stay away from foods that are known to you as allergens and these foods that are bad for everyone: white rice too often; white flour; animal fats or saturated fats; partially hydrogenated, hydrogenated fats; artificial sweeteners; processed foods; some chemicals; dye; artificial flavors; artificially and chemically made foods in a laboratory; some soft drinks; carbonated drinks; artificial salt and sodium; and outdated, expired, reduced, and contaminated foods. Be vigilant about what you eat, where you are, what you usually use, and what are new in your life. Be aware of changes in whatever you use. Because you can be using some cosmetics, detergents, cleaning products, food packages all your life and one day you pick up that product and have an allergic reaction. Why? Because something else is added or changed in that same products that you trust and omit to read the label. Do not confuse allergic reaction to sensitivity or intolerance. Sometimes some people have intolerance to milk or beans.

For milk, just use lactose-free milk and dairy products. For beans, to decrease flatulence, wash, soak in water, and refrigerate all beans the night before the last cooking steps. If that is the case, people won't have to stop using a food product.

Important Advice

Before I leave this chapter on allergy, I want to tell the readers that there is no need to spend a lot of money on doctor's bills and expensive tests and medications. I want the readers to know that in cases or conditions pertaining to allergy, people are their own best doctor, own expert investigator, and own lifesaver. Just tell your doctor about carrying a few capsules of over-the-counter Benadryl with you in your bag, pocket, and wallet. And whenever you feel the allergic symptoms or signs, place one of the capsules in your mouth with a sip of water from your bottle or any water within your reach until the signs or symptoms subside. Sometimes people only have signs that they don't even know or discover on their own. Signs like swelling, redness, and hives or urticaria without itching that can go unnoticeable to them until someone else asks them, "What happened to you?" or "Go look at yourself in a mirror!" Some other times the person affected would start itching and scratching from head to toe. Then this person is aware of the allergic reaction that can take too long for a doctor's visit. So this person needs to take his or her Benadryl, the brand name, or diphenhydramine hydrochloride (generic name) twenty-five-milligram capsule. If symptoms don't stop completely, this person at least has enough time to seek medical care.

There are signs and symptoms that people really need: a ready self-injected epinephrine pin or syringe before they end up with an anaphylactic shock. These signs and symptoms are chest pain, tingling in the mouth, swelling of the tongue, throat, difficulty breathing or shortness of breath, vomiting, or in extreme cases, loss of consciousness. The person then needs to self-inject his/her ready-to-use epinephrine, especially before going down to lose consciousness.

Something very important that people with known allergy to drugs and others things is to investigate about allergens in their life, making a list of known allergens and allergic reactions, give a copy to their doctor or doctors, discuss the list with them. They also need to carry that list with them at all times, make sure when they go to the hospital emergency department to show the list to the medical professionals, to the staff at the hospital. Write down or tell the staff about other allergens also besides drugs such as artificial sweeteners, iodine, dye, etc. that they are allergic to. Because for some tests, preps contain iodine, artificial sweeteners, contrast, etc. People should always carry a small notebook with a bright-red label saying, "I have a lot of allergies, and the list is inside this notebook to whom it may concern in case I lose consciousness." If you suspect food allergies, get tested. There is a cheap and painless skin-prick procedure that can be done at the doctor's office with immediate results that can provide an accurate diagnosis. After people know for sure all their food allergies besides not cooking these foods themselves, they need to make sure that they read labels of prepackaged foods. And if they have to eat at friends' or relatives' house, tell them about their food and ingredient allergies that can be in the meal preparations.

When people are eating out, they must give a call to inquire about the menu. And when they arrive at the place before they order their meals, they should inquire needed information from the person serving the foods or someone from the kitchen about foods and ingredients in the dishes. Allergic people should order their meals only if they are satisfied of all the answers concerning their foods and ingredients in preparation of all their meals.

Nevertheless, if people know that their allergic reactions are life-threatening, they should bring their self-injected epinephrine syringe or pin with them everywhere at all times. Remember, there is hope for allergy sufferers. Sometimes people with allergic reactions can stop and find themselves not allergic to some stuffs anymore and don't need to stop eating some foods they like safely. Unfortunately, sometimes people can acquire new allergies also and don't even know about them. But with their food diary, they can find out about new allergies and cut them out of their life or food supply. And if it is not possible for them to stay away from these new allergens, they just have to carry their Benadryl capsule or epinephrine syringe.

ALZHEIMER'S DISEASE

Alois Alzheimer was a German neurologist (1864 to 1915). Alzheimer's is a form of presenile dementia due to atrophy of the frontal and occipital lobes. It usually occurs between ages forty and sixty, more often in women than men. This condition involves progressive, irreversible loss of memory, deterioration of intellectual functions, apathy, speech and gait disturbances, and disorientation. Course may take from a few months to four or five years to progress to complete loss of intellectual function (Pick's disease).

Friedel Pick was a Czechoslovakian physician from 1867 to 1926 and who discovered non-rheumatic chronic pericarditis of unknown etiology.

Ludwig Pick, German physician (1868 to 1935), discovered Niemann-Pick disease.

Link between Cold Sores and Alzheimer's

If you are prone to cold sores, you may be at a higher risk for Alzheimer's disease, a new study shows. The virus that causes cold sores, herpes simplex virus 1, has also been found in Alzheimer's patients, leading doctors to believe it may play a role in the mind-destroying condition. Cold sores sufferers should be on the lookout for early signs of Alzheimer's and should inform their doctors immediately so that appropriate tests can be done. Dr. Ruth Itzhaki, who led the research team at Manchester University in England, predicts the discovery will lead to new treatments for Alzheimer's.

Boost Your Memory with Tasty New Diet

The diet favored by people who live on the shores of the Mediterranean Sea can improve your memory and cut your risk of getting Alzheimer's disease almost in half!

In the past, the diet has been touted as a delicious way to fight cancer and heart disease, but after the new study conducted at Columbia University in New York, scientists prove that the diet also promotes brain health.

Dr. Nikolaos Scarmeas and his colleagues studied the diets of 2,200 people older than age sixty-five and discovered that those who followed a Mediterranean-style food plan were 40 percent less likely to get Alzheimer's disease.

Dr. Marilyn Albert, a neurology professor at Johns Hopkins University and spokesperson for the Alzheimer Association, calls the research the most convincing evidence yet that plays a vital role in improving memory and preventing the tragic brain-destroying disease. The diet is easy to stick to. The principles are simple based on foods typically consumed by people living in Greece, Italy, and other Mediterranean countries.

The two main ingredients are olive oil and red wine. Other preferred foods are the following:

Eggplant
Tomatoes
Green and red peppers
Garlic
Oranges
Lentils
Dried beans
Onions
Fish/sardines
Whole-grain cereals and bread
Yogurt
Nuts with vitamin E that enhance memory
Zucchini
Chicory

Lemons
Bulgur wheat
Spinach
Artichokes and olives, which are powerful antioxidant
Leafy green vegetables

Blueberries contain a special type of antioxidant known to protect the brain from cell damage.

Cocoa boost brain power, so drinking a cup of cocoa a day can improve memory and mental alertness and protect people from brain diseases, such as dementia and Alzheimer's, said some researchers who presented their findings to a meeting of the American Association for the Advancement of Science. Cocoa contains special types of antioxidants called flavonoids that improve blood flow to the brain, said a doctor who studied the effects of the tasty drink using brain scans. Flavonoids appear to relax arteries, permitting better-sustained blood flow. The improved mental performance of all sorts is found in people who have cognitive impairment due to disease, brain damage, following a stroke or who are just fatigued and sleep deprived.

Herbs for Memory

There are some herbs that can greatly enhance people's ability to remember information at any age by including brain-boosting energy and clarity and that people should use in their daily diet. These natural products stimulate their brain cells and the processes by which those cells communicate with each other. These herbs are as follows:

Ginko biloba, which improves blood circulation to the brain. This keeps cells young and healthy, improving alertness and memory.

Hawthorn removes toxin from brain and strengthens blood vessels and tissue. It also helps brain cells utilize available oxygen.

Some other herbs that have demonstrated the ability to improve memory include gotu kola, bacopin (which also shorten learning time), rosemary, and schisandra.

Some foods to eat and drink in moderation:

Red meat, to be eaten in moderation like only 90 percent to 97 percent, fat-free lean steak or ground beef for making your own burgers once in a blue moon. Also, the meat has to be well protected, which you can learn how by reading the previous book T.H.A.T.S., The Health Assistance to Some. *Drink only 100 percent fruit juice three cups per week. Drink one to two glasses of alcoholic drinks once a month or only on special occasions. Eat only fat-free or reduced-fat dairy products. Drink only fat-free skimmed milk or reduced-fat milk. Don't forget to drink a lot of water seven to eight cups of eight ounces daily.*

Foods to Stay Away From

Stay away from foods containing saturated fats, hydrogenated fats, oil, or even partially hydrogenated fats, butter, fatty meats, and dairy products, white bleached flour baked goods with white sugar, white potatoes, white rice, white bread that is not made of whole grain, cereals, muffins, also.

Stay away from smoking and heavy alcoholic drinking. Don't be sedentary, exercise and move a lot, avoid elevators and escalators, walk and take the stairs, don't watch TV all day. Read books, magazines, and newspapers; watch only news and intellectual shows; play intellectual games; study; go to school; and socialize.

Some Tricks for Perfect Memory

How to Remember Names

Remember the names of new people you meet by writing them down, glancing at them before you go to bed that night, and your memory will retain them. Ask the person to repeat his name or say it, and you should call the person by his or her name right after that.

For Keys

Always drop your keys in the same place so you won't have to make a new mental note of where they are every time you put them down. This can be done for other objects also. I learned this one since I was a child from my father.

Directions

You can find easily where you are going by visualizing the journey before you set out, making a special note of landmarks that stand out.

Where You Parked Your Car

You will remember by turning around just after you lock the door and taking a mental snapshot of the area where you have left.

Situation

Recreate the situation just before you take the first step. The reason will flash into your mind immediately. Or go back where you came from, and while going back or returning, you will surely remember why you were there in the first place.

Let's go back to the Mediterranean diet with this one-day example. This diet is composed of so much vitamins, minerals, and fibers that doctors think it's a great diet for almost everyone, sick, old, to get better and younger and other to prevent diseases or conditions such as loss of memory and Alzheimer's. Some doctors believe that fish oil and vitamin C may be the components that lead to better memory and reduced risk of Alzheimer's. But the researchers stress that it's the combination of foods that's important and not just one or two elements.

A Typical Daily Menu

This typical daily menu that is based on the Mediterranean diet would look like this:

Breakfast

Small glass of four ounces of orange juice.

One slice of whole-wheat toast flavored with olive oil instead of butter.

One cup or six ounces of low-fat yogurt with a handful of almond or walnut mixed in it.

Morning Snack

A fruit if small, or a wedge of a large one.

Lunch

One eight-ounce cup of lentil soup.

A twelve-ounce bowl of salad made of spinach, lettuce, romaine preferred, radishes, and mushrooms with olive oil, herb-and-vinegar dressing.

One whole-wheat toast or small roll.

Afternoon Snack

One whole-wheat pita bread.

One tablespoon of hummus (a dip made from chickpeas that is available in most supermarkets or you can obtain the recipe and do it yourself from the T.H.A.T.S. Web site or anywhere else. Because it's better to cook your foods yourself so you will know for sure what's in your meals.

Dinner

One cup or two of whole-wheat pasta with sauce made with tomatoes, onions, garlic, green peppers, mushrooms, and zucchini.

One cup of white or red dried beans.

One moderate serving of fish, baked or grilled.

One small four-ounce glass of red wine for women and two for men.

Evening Snack

A handful of unsalted, roasted, or raw mixed nuts.

The key to success is to eat these Mediterranean foods every day, not just occasionally. Also limit your intake of red meat or other saturated fats to one or two servings every two weeks. Also limit your alcoholic intake to one to two small glasses once in a while because some doctors say that one glass of alcoholic beverage can be good for health, but too much alcohol can even cause Alzheimer's or loss of memory.

Other Ways to Promote Memory

New research proves that proper sleep is the most important factor in retaining information. Yet most Americans, particularly old citizens, suffer from serious sleep deprivation. While people are asleep, their brain cells remodel themselves, and failure to get the right amount of sleep causes symptoms similar to those associated with aging, including memory loss. Specifically, changes in glucose tolerance and endocrine function are noted in older people and in people of any age who don't get enough sleep.

Researchers suspect that chronic sleep loss may not only hasten the onset but could also increase the severity of age-related developments such as memory loss. Sleep plays a key role in the stabilization of memories. In a study conducted by Howard University professors in medicine and also experts in another university in Chicago, test subjects were asked to memorize a list of words at 9:00 AM. They were tested on how many of the words they could remember at nine o'clock that same evening and at nine the following morning.

On the evening test, they were able to remember 31 percent of the words, but in the morning test after a good night's sleep, they were able to recall 40 percent of them even though the second test was administered twelve hours after the first. The researcher speculates that during sleep, scattered thoughts are cleaned up and organized. Sleep might strengthen relevant associations, improving access to memories, said this researcher.

Additional studies have shown that the ability to remember both verbal and mathematical information drops dramatically in people who don't get adequate sleep. MRI scans detect less activity in the frontal cortex (the part of the brain that's involved in mathematical retention) and the left temporal lobe of the brain (which governs verbal retention) in sleep-deprived people.

Physiologically, information is first stored in a part of the brain called hippocampus. From there, it is transferred to the neocortex, where it is stored as memories. The transference occurs during sleep.

There are two types of sleep. Deep slow-wave sleep occurs at the beginning of the sleep cycle; light fast-wave sleep, also known as rapid-eye movement (REM) sleep, takes place toward the end. Both are important for memory retention.

During deep sleep, memories are consolidated in the hippocampus. Then during REM sleep, they are edited and transferred to the neocortex.

To get the right kind of sleep to boost memory function, you must follow certain steps:

1. *Go to bed only when you are tired and ready to fall asleep. Don't hit the sack if you are not feeling sleepy. You may drop off for an hour or two, but you will wake up too soon for proper REM sleep to occur.*
2. *Conversely, never stay awake past the point of tiredness. If you do, you will rob yourself of needed deep-wave sleep.*
3. *Try to wake up naturally without being jarred out of sleep by a jangling alarm clock. Give your natural sleep rhythm a chance to do its memory-enhancing work.*
4. *As you are falling asleep, review information that you want to remember so it will be available for transference from the hippocampus to the neocortex. Make note of important data during the day so you can go over them before bedtime.*

Too many people accept memory loss as an inevitable part of growing old. But experts and researchers have found that elderly brains are just as capable of learning and remembering as younger ones. And new brain cells and connections between brain cells can be developed at any age. In other words, there is no reason why you should ever forget anything again! In some most-read new books, scientists analyzed the most up-to-date research on memory loss, Alzheimer's disease, and dementia; and they have devised a simple five-step plan to banish the inconvenience, embarrassment, and anxiety of forgetfulness from your life.

The approach is straightforward, said these scientists in the book's guide to Alzheimer's disease, which should be mandatory reading for everyone older than fifty and anyone who fears that their memory lapses are symptoms of Alzheimer's disease and other forms of serious cognitive impairment. To me, the best way to keep your mind sharp is simply by exercising it just as with any regular physical activity, such as walking, which improves your heart and bring capacity to it, so mental activity can improve your brain function also. Give your brain a workout to keep it alert and energetic by staying in touch with family, friends, and coworkers and try to expand your circle of acquaintances. Go to movies, concerts, and plays. Read books, magazines, and newspapers. Do crossword puzzles. Take an adult education class, learn a craft. Do volunteer work. Stay up-to-date on current events and new technologies like computer and cell phones. If you don't have any reading material at all, learn ten new words a week from a dictionary and write yourself or a friend a letter using these new words.

This is the information age, and if you are not careful, you can end up buried in confusing piles of paper of varying degrees of importance. If you take time to notice how large your incoming mails are daily because of all the new advertising material that we never had before this age, you will see what I mean by age of information. In the mist of all the clutter, you may overlook or forget something really important. As solution, I suggest file instead of pile. Sort your mail as soon as it arrives. Make files for documents you will need to refer to later and throw the rest away immediately. And don't let junk accumulate.

Periodically, look over the file you have created and take out some papers, bank statements, credit card bills, supermarket receipts that you no longer need. Your goal is to keep clutter to a minimum. Make a daily to-do list and keep it in a prominent place, such as refrigerator door, top of your desk, or kitchen isle and countertop. Be sure to record appointments and tasks that must be done on that day and addresses and phone numbers relevant to that day's activities.

Have these three words in mind: routines, rituals, and cues. It's easier to remember to do things if you always do them in the same sequence or at the same time of the day and the same place wherever it is. For example, always keep your car keys in the same place or always shop on the same day of the week. I stick reminder notes in the same place, such as my refrigerator door, my bedroom mirror, top of my television, my desktop, at the side of my computer, etc., for different people as you wish.

Learn to develop a memory strategy. Whenever you learn something new, repeat the information several times to yourself. Associate the new information with similar facts you already know. Write the new data down on a piece of paper or a notebook, mention it in a conversation. Writing things down and saying them out loud are excellent ways to train your memory.

Take good care of your body. Your memory resides in your brain, and your brain is part of your body. Remember the old saying, "Sound mind in a sound body." So stay physically active, get plenty of sleep, limit alcohol consumption, quit smoking (you can do it), and try to manage stress. Also, antioxidants like vitamin E can prevent damage to brain cells, according to some researchers. Fruit juice can also decrease the risk of Alzheimer's. Some researchers say drinking two to three eight-ounce glasses of all-natural 100 percent fruit juice per week can prevent you from getting the disease. Better yet, get your fruits from the produce department organic and farm fresh. Wash them real well and drop them with peels, seeds, and water or skimmed milk in a food processor or blender with or without ice and drink it twice a week or even daily. If it can reduce the risk of having that dreaded mental disease, why not? According to statistics, more than 4.5 million Americans now suffer from Alzheimer's. That number is growing at an alarming rate every year and is expected to reach 16 million by the middle of the century. According to researchers, fruit juice could halt the horror in its tracks. It could prevent you from getting the disease, or if you are already at the early stage, ensure that you will not get worse. Fruit juice is better than fresh fruits because the chemicals that fight Alzheimer's are contained in the peel and pulp. Some of us, when we eat fresh fruits, often peel them first, but juice makers mash up the entire fruit in the manufacturing process, keeping the beneficial nutrients intact.

A study done by researchers at the Vanderbilt University in Nashville, Tennessee, tracked the health of two thousand people for ten years before releasing their findings in the prestigious American Journal of Medicine. *Lead researcher Dr. Qi Dai says, "We find that frequent drinking of fruit juices was associated with a substantially decreased risk of Alzheimer's disease." These findings are new and suggest that fruit juices may play an important role in delaying the onset of Alzheimer's.*

Alzheimer's expert Dr. Harriet Millward adds, "Diet could offer a relatively inexpensive way to fight a disease that ruins countless lives and costs more than cancer, stroke and heart disease put together."

Alzheimer's is caused by the accumulation of beta-amyloid protein in the brain. Antioxidants called polyphenols, abundantly available in the peel and pulp of certain fruits, can halt this buildup instantly. The most effective juices to drink to fight Alzheimer's are made from oranges, grapefruits, grapes, and apples. Vegetable juices also work. And fresh grapes and apples do the same if you eat them with the skin on.

Drinking three glasses of these fruit juices a week could mean that the disease can't fully take hold, says Dr. Ronald Petersen of the Mayo Clinic Alzheimer's Disease Center in Rochester, Minnesota.

Another study of 1,800 people by Dr. Amy Borenstein of the University of South Florida College of Public Health confirms the findings of the large study. She found that people who drank fruit or vegetable juice three times a week were four times less likely to develop Alzheimer's than those who drink little or no juice. Borenstein suggests a minimum of three eight-ounce glasses of juice per week.

More Good News on the Alzheimer's

There's more good news on the Alzheimer's front. Dr. Mark Sager of the University of Wisconsin Madison Medical School found that people who drink one to three alcoholic beverages a week also had a greatly reduced risk of Alzheimer's and memory loss in general. Red wine, which is especially rich in polyphenols, is the best drink to indulge in, he says.

Dr. Margaret Gatz of the University of Southern California adds that good dental health plays a role too. People with gum disease have a higher risk of Alzheimer's. So it's important to brush at least twice a day and floss your teeth at least once a day and see your dentist every six months for checkup and cleaning.

Staying mentally active by learning new skills and playing games like bingo and checkers, taking a daily walk, eating low-fat foods and whole grains, keeping your weight down can help a great deal in preventing memory loss and Alzheimer's.

Apples

I remember an advertisement for Kellogg's cereal in the mid sixties that goes like this: "New Kellogg's Apple Jacks a bowl a day keeps the bullies away." For other diseases, I say that an apple a day keeps the doctors away. But in Alzheimer's diseases, an apple a day may not keep the doctors away, it will help you remember your next appointment because apples improve memory for everyone at any age and fight Alzheimer's also, according to the following study.

A study done at the University of Massachusetts shows that apples contain a chemical that promotes the production of acetylcholine, a key brain neurotransmitter that improves memory and wards off all forms of dementia, including Alzheimer's disease. We anticipate that the day may come when foods like apples, apple juice, and other apple products are recommended along with the most popular Alzheimer's medications, says Dr. Thomas Shea, director of the University of Massachusetts Center for Cellular Neurobiology.

Many of the most promising Alzheimer's drugs on the market contain acetylcholine enhancers, says Dr. Thomas. People may ask, "What is acetylcholine?" Acetylcholine is an ester of choline occurring in various organs and tissues of the body. It is thought to play an important role in the transmission of nerve impulses at synapses and myoneural junctions. It is quickly destroyed by an enzyme, cholinesterase. Either excessive or deficient action of acetylcholine at the motor endplates may result in neuromuscular block.

Eye Test Spots Alzheimer's

An easy ten-minutes eye test can detect Alzheimer's disease before the first symptom manifests itself. If trial studies work out, it will be the first definitive method for determining the presence of the mind-wasting ailment and give doctors a chance to start treatment early enough to prolong high-quality life for their patients. The test, under development at Neuroptix company in Boston, is based on the finding that amyloid plaques, the cause of Alzheimer's, show up in the eyes before it appears in the brain.

A special drop that stains a type of protein that constitutes amyloid are put into the patient's eyes. The presence of the plaque then becomes simple to see under laser light. You probably ask yourself again, "What is amyloid?" This time, I am going to give you more information. Amyloid is a protein polysaccharide complex having starch-like characteristics produced and deposited in tissues during certain pathological states. It is a homogeneous, highly refractive substance staining readily with congo red. It is associated with a variety of chronic diseases, particularly tuberculosis, osteomyelitis, leprosy, Hodgkin's disease, and carcinoma.

According to this article of January 30, 2008, in ABC channel 7 news at 6:00 PM, scientists have found new treatment for Alzheimer's. Fifty deep brain stimulations, electrical pulses for electrical signal in obesity, has led them to serendipity finding for Alzheimer's (electrical devices implanted in the brain). Mild electrical current can spot memory was their findings. Some of their findings are that fish can reduce your chances of getting Alzheimer's disease by 40 percent. It's all due to the omega-3 fatty acids proven mood enhancers and brain boosters. Omega-3 fatty acids are in avocados, walnuts, almonds, flaxseed, and olive oil.

According to an article in Time *magazine page 25 of October 25, 2010, scientists claimed that the bleak landscape of Alzheimer's is changing for the past two years. Advances in a study of the human genome have opened up new avenues of exploration for Alzheimer's researchers in the realms of prevention and possible treatment. In this article, Patti Davis's father, former president Ronald Reagan, who died of Alzheimer's in 2004, and Maria Shriver's father, Sergeant Shriver, who was diagnosed with Alzheimer's in 2003, were mentioned. There was also a story on ABC's channel 7 reported by Christiane Amanpour on October 17, 2010, about Alzheimer's disease.*

Bottom line is, to prevent and help treat memory loss and Alzheimer's disease (adding to your medication), your diets, activities, and mental exercises are very important.

Foods

Forget about counting calories, holding on carbohydrate and good fats, this is not about weight loss. You need all food groups in this lifestyle diet.

Complex carbohydrates contain a vitamin that your gray matter in the brain needs to function better. This is vitamin B folic acid and could be found in whole grains, such as breads, cereals, pastas, and rice.

Good Fats

Fish oils from fish with omega-3 fatty acids like salmon, mackerel, sardine, olive oil, avocados, and some nuts are good fats that you need to be healthy in general.

Nuts contain vitamin E, which enhances memory. Green leafy vegetables like spinach, collard greens, kale, swish chard, and other greens contain vitamins that can help your memory. Fruits like apples, blueberries, and some others contain a special type of antioxidant that protects the brain cells from damage.

Habits and Techniques

Physical exercises: walk, pace, do head exercises, pushing and pulling and some low-impact exercise as you wish at your own pace, which are bicycling in or outdoor, stretching and flexibility exercises, swimming, water aerobics, deep-water walking, whatever you can do comfortably.

Mind exercises: reading, writing, studying, continuing education, learning to play a musical instrument, having a new habit, playing cards, chess, table games, puzzles, crosswords, finding words, spot-the-difference pictures, illusion confusion, etc., and pay attention to what is going on around you.

Reward more instead of punish.
Look at the good more instead of the bad.
See the positives more instead of the negatives.
Remember the good instead of the bad.
Forget the bad and the negatives instead of remembering them.

When you find one good and positive quality in something or someone, emphasize it, reward it, give recognition to it, and share it with others. Be generous with the good and compassionate with the bad and the ugly and imperfect.

Do not stay in the past mistakes and deal with regrets, grudges, revenge, and hate.

It is better, faster, and more rewarding to forget, forgive, and move on with love, good deeds, happiness, creativity, risk taking, new creations, activities, new ideas, and learning better-coping skills to correct past mistakes and enjoy greater accomplishment.

Erase old learning and replace them with new ones because your brain and memories are like an old tape recorder and cassette. Sometimes when the cassettes are full, you tend to record on them over and over until they become ineffective and too crowded. Then you need to erase some old information and replace them with new ones. Especially with new technology such as the CD, iPod, cell phones, computer, e-mail, Internet. If you are an older person, you have your work cut out for you to be able to function adequately at the present.

Your brain or mind is like a house that you continuously add furniture, papers, documents, bills, magazines, advertisements, flyers, and pamphlets to. Therefore, you have to assess, sort, and organize them to see what you can get rid of and declutter the house. You have to do the same with the bad-spirited attitudes, information, and feelings and replace them with good, positive, generous, happy, giving, and wonderful humanitarian information and actions that you can share with others way before you have Alzheimer's or you might never have it at all if you have been this changed admirable human being after reading this chapter.

Alzheimer's is not just one disease caused by one thing, such as genes or heredity or bad nutrition, or smoking, drinking, overweight, lack of sleep, or lack of activity. Alzheimer's is a process that needs a lifestyle change for the better before it gets too far. Genes or heredity is just 20 percent in the process, which can be defeated with the 80 percent boost from a new lifestyle change, adding to all new techniques and advices in this chapter.

Know What to Decrease

Decrease stress, anxiety, animosity, fear, argument, hate, and aggression. These are cause of many diseases and conditions, including Alzheimer's, which will become epidemic in this country just like obesity, diabetes, hypertension, cholesterol (fatty LDL). With all the above, no wonder the brain shuts down and can no longer cope. The brain says, "Enough is enough." Therefore, instead of manic depressive, bipolar, chronic undifferentiated, schizophrenic, schizoaffective, which we have before, is changed now to psychopath, dementia, Alzheimer's, ADHD (hyperactive) and aggressive people in all class, race, and age group.

Summary for Alzheimer's

At the Institute for Biological Studies in California, scientists found out that physical exercise builds brain cells and could help old people stay sharp and mentally alert all through their lives. Contrary to common belief, exercise is not only for young people. Exercise can benefit people at any age. Scientists confirm in the same studies that exercise can help prevent and replace damaged gray matter, causing the brain-destroying disease like Alzheimer's.

Therefore, why not start to exercise at any age? Better yet, why not lift weight at home, such as five, eight, and ten pounds of dumbbell on each hand up and down and barbells twenty-five to fifty pounds at home or at a gym to start with our feet. If possible, have a coach tell you what is the best for your age. If you can't do any of these, walk briskly or at your own pace for a half hour daily or at least five days a week. Pacing and stair climbing can be done at home if you can't go outside. It's a must that you keep moving and sit down the least as possible. Play a sport if you can at any age; it's good and benefits the brain besides muscle, mood, and spirit. Know that physical exercise can build brain cells and help old people stay sharp for the rest of their lives. Brain-building power of exercise is not only for young people. Several scientific studies show that old people benefit greatly by pumping iron or lifting weight and hope to get rid of brain-destroying diseases like Alzheimer's, dementia, and replace damaged gray matter.

Foods for Memory

Eat foods that can boost your memory and help you grow new and healthy brain cells to prevent memory loss and promote a perfect memory. Foods that contain B vitamins boost brain power. Two of the vitamins B, B12, and folate can improve memory and mental functions in older people, according to a study. Many old American people suffer from deficiency of the vitamin B12. Fortunately, there are a lot of foods in this country that can provide vitamin B12 and folate. In the food chapter in this book Food for Health and Cure, *there is a list of foods to add to your diet for almost every condition or disease to help people in need. Some foods that contain vitamin B12 are meat, poultry, eggs, and dairy products. And foods that contain folic acid are leafy vegetables, citrus fruit, and dried beans of all types and color. Other good foods are whole grains, bread, and cereals.*

Fish: salmon, mackerel and sardines.

Leafy vegetables: spinach, chickory, kale, collard greens, mustard green, etc.

Nuts also are good for everyone and mostly for people with Alzheimer's because they are loaded with vitamin E, which is a memory enhancer.

Some Tricks to Help Memory

Always drop your keys or eyeglasses at the same place at all times.

Write down the names of the people you just meet. Before writing the name, ask the person, "What is your name please?" Repeat the name aloud until you finish writing it down.

Write down directions, visualize the landmarks, see the trips back and forth, including the signs and traffic lights, and count them.

To remember where you park your car, turn around make a mental picture of the area, write down in your address book or a piece of paper from your pocket or purse the address, the name of the cross streets, the lot number before you leave the car and the place.

If you happen to walk upstairs or away from where you were and forget why you did that in the first place, in this situation, go back down or where you were and recreate the situation. Just before you take the first step, the reason will flash into your mind right away.

Do crossword puzzles, secret-word puzzles, and picture puzzles, word games or any game that can make your memory and brain sharper. Just do them preferably during the day and not at night or not too close to bedtime or sleeping time. Because they will keep you awake.

And remember not to ever rely on your memory alone no matter how old you are. Write down information, take notes, make videos, take pictures, record information on tape, keep some of your special occasions pictures and cards, and save them somewhere that you can find them at a glance. I guarantee you that there will come a time that you will be listening, looking at or reading something that you couldn't believe you did. I learned that from my father as a child, from some of my teachers in almost every degree I own, especially psychology, nursing, and education.

For this reason, I write letters to my children, my husband, my friends, or to my coworkers and always make a copy for myself. Sometimes I send the letters or notes and keep the copies. Other times, I don't send them at all and keep both for many years and get a good surprise. It's always something that changes meanings or thinking or writing ability to me. It's even better than a diary to me because you can say more in a letter than a diary. If I want to go back in time, I can just open the box and read one or two of my letters or open a family album and look at old pictures and be happy, or solve a problem that I did not see before and hope for the better. In bad times, this helped me to appreciate, work harder for something, have courage to perseverate, fight for according to which letter I open and read. The above can prevent loneliness, keep you busy, jolt your memory, and prevent diseases like Alzheimer's.

ANEMIA

Anemia is either not enough red blood cells or hemoglobin in the blood. This results in the amount of oxygen that the blood is able to carry. Anemia decreases the amount of oxygen in the cells of the body. The result is less energy to perform normal functions. Important processes like muscular activities, cell repair and building become slower and less efficient. If the brain lacks oxygen, dizziness may occur and mental faculties are less sharp.

What Is Anemia?

Anemia itself is not a disease, but only a symptom of many diseases. Any deficient production of red blood cells or destruction of red blood cells can turn to anemia. Anemia can be the first sign for many diseases, conditions, and disorders. It is sometimes the first sign detected in arthritis, some other major diseases, cancer, drug use, hormonal disorders, chronic inflammation in the body, surgery, infections, peptic ulcers, hemorrhoids, diverticulosis, or diverticulitis, heavy menstrual bleeding, numerous pregnancies, liver damage, thyroid disorders, rheumatoid arthritis, bone marrow disease, dietary deficiencies such as iron, folic acid, vitamins B6 and B12 can all cause anemia. Hereditary diseases, like sickle cell and thalassemia, can cause anemia. In the United States of America, according to statistics, about 71,000 people are affected with these diseases. These people are of African American and Mediterranean descent.

Thalassemia

This is a group of hereditary anemias occurring in populations bordering the Mediterranean and in Southeast Asia. This type of anemia is produced by either a defective production rate of the alpha or beta hemoglobin polypeptide chain or a decrease synthesis of the beta chain. Heterozygotes are usually asymptomatic. The severity in homozygotes varies according to the complexity of the inheritance patterns, but may be fatal sometimes.

Sickle-Cell Anemia

Sickle cell is an abnormal red blood corpuscle that has a crescent shape. Sickle-cell anemia is a hereditary chronic form of anemia in which abnormal sickle or crescent-shaped erythrocytes are present. Due to the presence of abnormal type of hemoglobin, hemoglobin S in the red blood cells shows. High occurrences of this disease are in Mediterranean and African populations.

Blood Tests

In a blood test called CBC with differential (complete blood count), the result shows anemia when hemoglobin content is less than 13 to 14 gram per 100 milliliter for males or 11 to 12 gram per 100 milliliter for females. If the beginning of the anemia is slow, the body may adjust so well that there will be no functional impairment though the hemoglobin may be less than 6 gram per 100 milliliter of blood, meaning that the person with anemia may be working, talking, or dancing with you and suddenly will collapse in front of your eyes without warning.

There are other ways to detect anemia from a blood test, which are on the basis of mean corpuscular volume (MCV) as microcytic less than 80 not enough or too little. Normocytic more than 80 to 94 is normal, normal in size, and more than that number is macrocytic, too much or too big cells. MCH hypochromic is less than 27; 27 to 32 normochromic means that your blood cells are normal in size, and more than 32, the cells are too big.

And last by etiological factors. Anemia can result from large amounts of blood loss and large amounts of blood cell destruction or decrease of blood cell formation. Anemia caused by blood loss is usually because of acute or chronic hemorrhage. Anemia due to blood cell destruction occurs in hemolytic diseases or hypersplenism.

TREATMENT

Consume foods with iron, vitamin B12, folic acid, ascorbic acid, rest to increase energy, sleep for seven to eight hours per night. Drink seven to eight eight-ounce cups of spring water. Take good care of your skin, mouth, teeth, and gums, have a good lifestyle change, and stop smoking, using drugs, and alcohol drinking. Have a good diet rich in fresh fruits, vegetables, nuts, whole grains, and lean protein. Some of the fruits are oranges, grapefruits, tangerines, peaches, pears, berries, apples, pineapples, grapes, melons, tomatoes, cantaloupes, mangoes, avocados, and dried fruits such as raisins, figs, and dried prunes.

The vegetables are beets, kale, chards, collard greens, carrots, watercress, celery, cabbages of all colors, green pepper and all the colors of pepper, onions, broccoli, sweet potato, other colors of potato, green plantains, and many more. Eat all types of whole grains as fortified cereal, breads, rice of all color and little of white rice, pastas of whole grains.

Protein: foods with iron beef and calf liver, lean beef steak, burgers, poultry, fish, and low-fat dairies. First find out what type of anemia you have and what diet is appropriate for you because in some cases, iron is bad and in others, iron is the best.

Anemia due to decreased blood formation may result from defective nucleoprotein synthesis (such as pernicious and other macrocytic anemia), deficiency of iron in the diet, inhibition of bone marrow (as in certain toxic states), loss of bone marrow or bone marrow failure.

Most of the time, people with anemia are treated with iron pills, vitamins, liver extract, B-complex over the counter, vitamin supplements or with eating their own food containing the vitamins needed.

SYMPTOMS

Some symptoms of anemia are skin pallor, no blood color under the fingernail beds when you press the nails down, pale color of mucous membranes, general weakness, vertigo, headache, sore tongue, drowsiness, general malaise, dyspnea, tachycardia (rapid pulse or heartbeat) palpitation (fast and shallow heartbeat, angina pectoris (a heart condition), gastrointestinal problems, amenorrhea (no menstruation), loss of libido (no sexual desire), and light fever.

Sometimes and in some cases of anemia, bed rest is recommended by your doctor. If not, continue your daily activities and some non-strenuous exercises, such as walking and stretching.

ANOREXIA NERVOSA

Anorexia nervosa is a loss of appetite seen in depression, start malaise, fevers, and some illnesses. Sometimes it happens because of disorders of the alimentary tract, such as the stomach; alcoholic excesses; and drug addiction, especially cocaine.

This loss of appetite for food can't be explained as a local disease. So far, nervosa is a complex condition that is poorly understood. It usually appears to be a symptom of mental illness. Females from age twelve to twenty-one years old are the most affected by this disease. Sometimes older women and a few men can have it also.

The symptom is not associated with specific neurosis or psychosis. A progressive severe loss of weight and amenorrhea in women (loss of menstruation) and impotence in men may happen.

In young children, it is one of the few psychiatric disorders that may lead to death. The person denies that anything is wrong even when emaciated. In some cases, the person having this disorder must be hospitalized to receive psychiatric therapy. If this person refuses to eat, he or she must receive tube feeding.

If the person can eat, encourage instead of forcing. Reward and don't punish. Encourage him or her to sit with other people for meals. Make meals appetizing by using spices and colorful herbs. Decorate the table like a personal holiday to this person. Play music that the person likes. Don't talk, but acknowledge with nonverbal behavior with some "uhmm, ahahaha!" And do this with a head shake up and down and a wide smile of approval. Pay close attention to this person. Even if the person eats just a little, don't say anything negative; accept it and hope for better next time. Also, tell these people right away, "You did fine for this time, next time will be much better." Don't forget to give the person a token of appreciation, such as something that he or she likes and for you not to go too far out of your way. This act can promote positive reinforcement.

GOOD FOODS

Good foods for people affected with this disease are as follows:

Double and triple protein meals so that all the protein allowance for the day can be consumed in a small portion of the meals.

EXAMPLES

Breakfast

Eggs, cheese, milk and toasts. Make an omelet with the three proteins on top of a half toast.

Two types of cheese, one slice of bread to make a grilled cheese sandwich with four ounce of milkshake with whole milk and powdered milk.

Egg, whole milk, and fortified plant protein whole-grain cereal for cooked or dry, cold cereal.

Lunch

Mixed garden salad with nuts, chicken pieces, and cheese for three proteins; romaine lettuce, cucumber, carrot, radishes, and homemade salad dressing with milk, olive oil, colorful pieces of olive.

Make cakes, cookies, rolls, and croissants with beans, cheese, meat, poultry, fish, seafood, whole-grain pastas, brown rice, and other pastries. Make them small and tasty but powerful with vitamins, minerals, and combined proteins. Make balls of peanut butter and jelly and desserts and pastries with fresh and dry fruits, ice cream in colorful cones or decorated glasses. Don't worry about using salt and sugar with some saturated fats in this person's meals. Don't use trans fat and high-fructose corn syrup in this person's diet.

Don't make or give a simple meal for this person. Make and give complicated, exotic, colorful, and attractive dishes with almost all food groups for the individual to consume all the vitamins, minerals, hormones, and enzymes needed.

Do not hide to put any nutrient powders or crushed vitamin pills, tablets, or liquid syrup. If you do these tricks, you are done. He or she wouldn't trust you and wouldn't eat nor drink from you or anyone else. He or she will rather die of hunger than eat or drink from someone. Don't forget that people afflicted by this disease still have a keen sense of smell and taste.

They can distinguish what are natural or man-made and artificial foods or drugs; adding to it the lack of trust anyway.

When dealing with people affected with anorexia nervosa or just plain anorexia, don't blame and don't make negative remarks or criticisms pertaining to the disease. Treat them as normal and regular individuals, entertain them, listen to music, watch lively, funny shows and movies, play games that are easy, joke and laugh a lot around them. Feed them natural, organic, and fresh foods at all times.

ANXIETY

Sometimes anxiety is demonstrated in apprehension, restlessness, tiredness, and your legs and toes will start twitching. Other times, anxiety gives you a feeling of apprehension, worry, uneasiness, or dread of the future. If it is just boredom or loneliness, just get dressed and go out for a walk where you can meet and see and talk to people.

Everyone has been anxious and will be anxious at some time. People are anxious, especially close to final exams, end of semester exams in school, college entrance exams, presentations, graduations, board exams, bar exams, job exams, starting new jobs, moving in a new place, going on a date, etc. Almost any normal circumstance in life can produce anxiety.

Anxiety is the normal reaction to that which is threatening to one's body, lifestyles, values, and loved ones relationships. Being in love and someone loving you can promote anxiety. Certain amount or degrees of anxiety is normal and stimulates the person's purposeful action. As a matter of fact, psychology encourages a little anxiety in everything in our life to be meaningful. What is neither good nor beneficial (as in everything in life) is excess anxiety. Excessive anxiety interferes with efficient functioning of anyone. Excess anxiety is bad, so bad that it's not anxiety anymore. It turns to psychosis or neurosis.

ANXIETY NEUROSIS

This is a mental disorder with characteristics of anxiety to excess, which is not restricted to specific situations or objects. And it is also associated with somatic symptoms or complaints. This disorder must be differentiated from normal anxiety, which occurs in realistically threatening situations.

Anxiety neurosis may be manifested when a person without organic disease during clear consciousness complains of palpitation; heart pain; dyspepsia; cold, sweaty, tremulous extremity; constriction of the throat; or pressure about the head. Very often, these symptoms are misinterpreted as meaning regional disease.

TREATMENT

Investigate and find out what causes this condition. Most of the time, it happens to people faced with stressful situations. The situations are economical, dysfunctional family, marital problems, quarrel, domestic violence, feeling of being trapped in desperate situations for too long where the person can no longer see the light at the end of the tunnel. The mind or brain develops some kind of defense mechanism to help the affected person cope until something good happens to save him or her. Sometimes, the doctor's visits, the all-negative tests and normal vital signs, no prescription for drugs can be the beginning of something positive for the individual. The rest are meeting new compassionate people, forming new interesting relationships, change in better treatments, laughter, enjoyment, fun, a good-paying job, a sense of purpose by doing something the person really likes can progress to a new beginning for the individual. Later on, if the individual still has some free time, he or she can get involved in a charitable group or institution, learn a foreign language, a new dance, or any other hobby. The most important part of the treatment is a lifestyle change by cutting all bad habits, such as smoking, drinking alcoholic beverages excessively instead of one daily four ounces of any alcoholic drink for women and two for men or eight ounces of beer for women and two eight-ounce cans or glasses or bottles for men. Other things to stay away from are taking drugs, eating bad foods, fast-foods, junk foods, fried foods, poorly prepared foods, and processed foods with high-fructose corn syrup, hydrogenated, partially hydrogenated, or trans fat.

People affected by neurosis should eat all-natural, organic, fresh, nutritious foods of all groups in the pyramid, such as complex carbohydrates: breads, grains, cereal, brown rice, pasta, whole grains, and wheat. Eat fresh fruits, vegetables, salad of all colors. Eat fish, lean beef, poultry, low-fat or fat-free organic dairy products, nuts, seeds, and good fats like flaxseed, olive oil, avocado, dark chocolate, and peanut butter. Since anxiety is associated with stress that makes people grumpy, crabby, cranky, and in foul mood, let us feed them with some good-mood food to make them laugh and boost their energy.

These foods are the following:

Complex carbohydrate that produces an amino acid called tryptophan, which tells the brain to make serotonin, one of the feel-good (hormone) chemicals that calm you down like a tranquilizer. Whole-grain cereals hot and cold, old-fashioned oatmeal for breakfast with low-fat or fat-free milk, one-half of a large banana or a whole small banana for potassium, a calming mineral.

Spinach and other dark green leafy vegetables that contain folate, a B vitamin that helps the production of serotonin again. Spinach also contains a mineral named magnesium that can raise your mood, lower your nervous system, regulate depression, anxiety, and increase your energy.

Fruits can do the trick too because of their natural sugar that can raise glucose that the brain needs to function properly. Sometimes a few plantain chips with 2 percent sodium or a few homemade sweet potato chips can help also due to the salt content or sodium that our brain and body needs in small amounts to function properly and raise our mood.

Dairy products like a cup or glass of milk hot or cold, a glass or cup of dark chocolate with organic low-fat or fat-free milk can calm your nerve and help you sleep because of the tryptophan and serotonin that can reduce your anxiety level, irritability, frustration, anger, and increase your energy and good mood. Milk has a mineral named calcium that can relax your muscles, balance your blood pressure, and strengthen your bones besides increasing your laughter.

Remember to eat a well-balanced meal every four to five hours at the most. Eat a snack of fruits, nuts, and chips as needed two to three hours between meals or as a meal replacement. Drink six to eight eight-ounce glass or cup of *spring water before, between, and after meals. Also, you need to have a good seven to eight hours of sleep every night. All the above can prevent the ups and downs in your blood sugar that can have an impact on your well-being.*

Make Some Comfort Foods

Macaroni and cheese: make it your own way by using these ingredients: whole-wheat macaroni of your choice, fat-free organic fresh milk or 2 percent at the most, margarine with vegetable oil (no trans fat) or natural butter, fat-free ricotta cheese, grated hard cheese, onion, garlic powder or fresh, a dash of salt and black pepper, or any other seasoning of your choice without MSG.

Make soup with dried beans of any color; add carrots, celery, green and red bell pepper, chickpeas, and chicken breast. Cut sweet potato in big chunks with skin, sprinkle season of your choice and olive oil, and bake on cookie sheet in the oven. Eat a chocolate cookie once a week as dessert or snack, and eat dry black beans with brown rice. Just know that you have to fight for yourself to stay above the hole, heal yourself, and win the fight.

When you feel stressed out, overwhelmed with anxiety, close to high anxiety, do the following:

Slow down in everything, such as talking slowly, moving slowly, walking slowly, eating slowly, and breathing slowly and deeply. In a few minutes after slowing down your pace, you will find out that you are thinking more clearly, reacting more reasonably and more appropriately to people and situations or whatever it is that caused your stress and anxiety. Anxious people are also stressed-out people. Usually, they tend to speak fast and breathlessly. By slowing their body down, they will surely regain control over almost any situation.

When you feel overwhelmed, call a friend. But it has to be someone that you know for sure can put a smile on your face instead of unloading his or her problems, more stress and anxiety on you, and turn out to be a stressor for more anxiety. Talking to a friend that is gentle, understanding, and a good listener can help your health mentally, spiritually, emotionally, and physically.

Meditation and Imagery

At any time, day and night, take five to ten minutes even twenty minutes (depending on where you are) to meditate. It can be at work by your desk. Just close your eyes or leave them open, but close your mind and relax for five minutes, take five deep breaths slowly through your nose, bring the air all the way down to your belly, saying, "Hummmm," holding it as long as you can and exhaling it out through your mouth very slowly. At home, go to a quite room with no light and sit down or lie down. Whatever you chose, take fifteen to twenty minutes doing it. Next, picture yourself in a place that you were happy and comfortable, laughing with loved ones or doing anything enjoyable.

Doing the above can help you release less of the "fight and fly" hormone named cortisol, which releases high anxiety and stress level. Some more advice about fighting anxiety and stress: Dress down sometimes, wear an old outfit instead of shopping for new clothes for every occasion. Wear wigs sometimes instead of going to the beauty salon every two weeks. You can also wash your hair, blow-dry, and roll it or make a ponytail yourself. Cook your meals at home and bring your lunch and snacks from home in a T.H.A.T.S. REFRIGERATOR COOLER BAG, which you can purchase online at the Web site mariethats.com or you can buy your own bag and add ice pack in it to protect your food. Get a lower-paying job that is long-term, steady with benefits, instead of a high-paying but stressful one. The bottom line is in order to decrease anxiety, you have to get rid of stress.

ARTERIOSCLEROSIS

This is applied to many pathological conditions when there is thickening, hardening, and loss of elasticity of the walls of the arteries; the above results in altered function of tissues and organs. Changes can occur in the intima, the media, or in both.

Some types of Arteriosclerosis

Medial: the medial is arteriosclerosis of the peripheral arteries that contain calcium deposits in the media.

Nodular: the nodular is arteriosclerosis from fibrous plaques in the intima.

Obliteran: the obliteran is the arteriosclerosis that closes the lumen of the arteries completely.

Senile: the senile is arteriosclerosis caused by old age.

Arteriosclerosis can be caused by untreated high blood pressure or hypertension.

According to scientists, the cause or origin of arteriosclerosis is unknown. It appeared to be caused by aging, altered lipids, metabolism, factors in the environment, chemicals, psychological, physiological, and genetic elements. All the above can contribute to arteriosclerosis. We know that some risk factors—such as hypertension, increased blood lipids, especially cholesterol and triglycerides, obesity, diabetes mellitus, inability to cope with stress, anxiety, family history of the disease, and physical inactivity—can lead to the disease. We also know that more males than the female sex at the age of thirty-five to forty-four years old and in general die of this disease. And white male death rate is six times that of white females.

TREATMENT

Activity

Regular activities, exercise, walking, jogging, pacing, running, mowing lawns, shoveling snow, raking leaves, cleaning your house, washing your dishes and your clothes by hand can help a great deal.

Socialization

Dance with a partner in a nightclub or at home by yourself, laugh, have fun, play a sport with friends and relatives, play table games, have a good support system and effective coping skills. Avoid anxiety and stress. Diet or normal food intake. Eat fresh produce, organic green leafy vegetables cooked by you at home. Eat fresh organic fruits like kiwi, cherries, apples, bananas, oranges, grapefruits, melons, cantaloupe, pineapples, honeydew, berries, tomatoes, avocados, red grapes, and nuts, especially wall nuts and brazil nuts to lower your cholesterol fatty LDL and raise good cholesterol HDL and decrease your blood pressure also.

Grains

Eat brown rice, oatmeal, whole-wheat bread and pasta and bran fiber food, cereal, and other products containing whole grains and whole wheat.

STAY AWAY

Stay away from stress, sitting down for too long; when sitting, get up every two hours and walk around for ten minutes at least. Avoid a sedentary lifestyle, fast-foods, salty foods, saturated fats or animal fat, hydrogenated fats, partially hydrogenated fats or trans fats. Don't drink soft drink with high-fructose corn syrup, sugar, salt, sodium, and carbonated. Don't eat foods made with white bleached flour, white rice, white potatoes, and fat dairy products such as butter, milk, yogurt, cream and cheese that's not fat free or 1 to 2 percent fat-free and 2 to 4 percent sodium. Read labels before you buy and consume any food.

Avoid Conditions

Avoid all conditions that can increase your blood pressure. Know that the lower your blood pressure is, the better for you. Your blood pressure goes according to your age, sex, race, and family history. The normal blood pressure is usually 120/80, but if yours is lower down to 110/70 or in between, it is even better if you are an adult and older; people can have it up to 130/85, but with a diastolic or lower number less than 90 is still good.

If you already know that you have arteriosclerosis, do not apply hot water bottles or compresses, heat pads, or any type of heat to your arms and legs or any parts of your body. Sometimes it's better to stay in bed, avoid stress, anxiety, and physical activities until your condition ameliorates. And please do not smoke, drink alcoholic beverages, and use drugs that are not prescribed by your doctors. Have yearly or semiannual checkups by your cardiologist, your primary doctors, and keep your appointments up-to-date.

ARTHRITIS

Arthritis is a chronic systemic condition. Arthritis is an inflammation of a joint, usually accompanied by pain and sometimes change in structure.

Arthritis may result from or be associated with many conditions including infections such as gonococcal, tuberculous, pneumococcal, rheumatic fever, ulcerative colitis, trauma, neurogenic disturbances as tabes dorsalis, degenerative joint disease as osteoarthritis, metabolic disturbances as gout, neoplasms as synovioma, hydrarthrosis, para or periarticular conditions as fibromyositis, myositis, or bursitis, various other conditions as acromegaly, psoriasis, Raynaud's disease.

Acute Secondary Arthritis

Acute secondary arthritis caused by osteitis have symptoms that are severe pain, redness, and swelling. People can have other rare forms of arthritis, such as acute suppurative arthritis, which is a purulent distention of the synovial sac. It's a dangerous form of arthritis.

Allergic Arthritis

Another neglected form of arthritis is the allergy that appears after eating food allergens or occurring in serum sickness. That means you eat some foods, don't know that you are allergic to them, don't react the common way like itching, sneezing, running nose, teary eyes. Instead, you have pain in your knees, joints, arms, fingers, and neck.

Gonorrheal Arthritis

Gonorrheal arthritis is due to gonorrheal infection. It usually causes pain in the knee joints during acute stage, meaning at the beginning. Later on, many other joints may be affected also. For this type of arthritis, if diagnosed, antibiotics should be given by your doctor besides eating good foods, applying hot and cold compresses, and practicing mild exercises.

Osteoarthritis

It is a chronic disease involving the joints those bearing weight. This type of arthritis is characterized by degeneration of articular cartilage, overgrowth of bones with lipping and spur formation, and impaired function or degenerative joint-disease hypertrophic.

Rheumatoid Arthritis

It is a chronic systemic disease characterized by inflammatory changes in joints and related structures that result in crippling deformities. What causes it is unknown. But it's believed that the pathological changes in the joints are related to an antigen-antibody reaction, which is poorly understood. Environmental and familial factors are in doubt. People usually have this disease by the middle ages and rarely at any age.

There is no specific treatment. For a lot of pain, bed rest is required for a short period of time. Salicylate, for example, aspirin and sodium salicylate, are used. Anti-inflammatory agents like indomethacin, ibuprofen, corticosteroids are used for acute inflammation when prescribed by your doctor, besides home remedies, good habits, good foods, and exercises. Any local treatment is used for a short time for acute pain and not for cure or prevention. Exercise, physiotherapy, and maintaining range of motion of affected joints are important to prevent contracture and promote mobility and flexibility. When the pain and swelling or inflammation decreases, active exercise is used to promote muscle strength and range of motion. A large amount of self-help devices are available in the market for afflicted people to remain self-sufficient. In severe cases, surgical procedures such as total hip replacement and arthroplasty are used with good results for people affected with this form of arthritis.

STATISTICS

According to statistics of 2006, in the United States alone, there are 36 million Americans who suffer from arthritis. Some have severe inflammation of the joints, stiffness, swelling, redness, limited mobility and range of motion. That means they can't move some of their body parts the way they want to. These people are in pain most of the time. Later on, they have fever, fatigue, insomnia, and problem breathing. Their cartilage and other tissues that hold the joints together are damaged and deformed. Sometimes some people can't walk or do other daily activities because of so much stiffness and pain. For some people who are obese or overweight, it is double trouble. Therefore, it is recommended by scientists and me that everybody in general lose weight before they have arthritis. And while they are already suffering from it, losing weight is imperative to decrease pain and suffering.

Defense against Arthritis

Defense against arthritis, one of the diseases plaguing Americans in our time, is an important knowledge. In this book, you will find a lot of techniques, good habits, fun things to do, good foods to eat, herbal tea and drinks to drink, home remedies and exercises to help decrease, stop, and eliminate for good all suffering. Before you take a pill that can make you sick, give you side effects and addiction, and can even kill you sometimes, try to use or do what is in this chapter.

Pumpkin seeds stop arthritis pain in its tracks! The tasty seeds are loaded with zinc, an important nutrient that build cartilage and ligaments and strengthens muscles. The seeds also contain essential fatty acids, which reduce inflammation and alleviate pain.

In a recent study, pumpkin seeds performed as well as some arthritis drugs, such as Indomethacin (Indocin) with none of the medicine side effects, no headaches, no dizziness, and no insomnia and diarrhea.

The first thing that I will suggest is to lose weight to decrease your arthritis pain. For every pound of body weight, your hips and knees feel fifteen to ten pounds of pressure, according to me and some other scientists. If you are obese, you will look like and feel like an eight-wheeler tractor trailer on top of a Volkswagen Beetle with four little tires, meaning that all your top parts are going to crash down on your bottom parts, starting from your lower back, hips, knees, ankles, heels, and feet, leaving you screaming in pain. Therefore, lose ten to fifty pounds, depending on how much you weigh and free yourself from pain.

According to a scientific research, apple cider vinegar and garlic can relieve the pain from arthritis. What you do is chop and grind one clove of fresh garlic or half of a teaspoon of garlic powder (no salt), mix it with two teaspoons of apple cider vinegar in an eight-ounce glass of warm temperature water and drink it once for the day that you have pain for immediate relief.

Other foods that are good to relieve pain are: all berries, all tomatoes, all oranges, grapefruits, cabbages, broccoli, regardless of colors, and cauliflower. Because these foods are anti-inflammatory and pain is usually caused by inflammation of the nerves. These foods are also antioxidants.

Other groups of foods that can decrease pain because they contain omega-3 fatty acids are salmon, mackerel, tuna, sardine, eggs, flaxseed, brazil nuts, hazelnuts, pecans, walnuts, and spinach.

Foods that contain flavonoids and are good for pain relief also are green tea, onions, soy and their products, grapes, and apples.

Foods with resveratrol are good for pain relief, like berries, peanuts, and peanut butter.

Foods with beta-cryptoxanthin that are good to relieve pain are watercress, watermelon, plums, tangerines, peaches, nectarines, bell peppers of all colors, and apricot.

According to my own experience and scientists, these roots and spices are also good for pain: ginger root, my favorite number one remedy, followed by bromelain, ginseng, licorice, cat's claw, echinacea, turmeric, skullcap, yucca, and many more. For me, since it's mind over matter, meditation, imagery, hypnosis, and biofeedback help a lot for various types of pain. I usually leave medication for last resort and only if I must because of side effects of any kind coming from medications that I don't like.

Other foods that can provide relief from arthritis pain because they contain minerals are zinc, magnesium, copper, and also an enzyme called superoxide. This enzyme is in the inflamed joints where it neutralizes free radicals. Zinc is in many enzymes that can decrease arthritis pain.

The foods that contain zinc and copper that can fight inflammation in the joints are poultry, lean meat, beef, chicken, lamb, goat, turkey, crabmeat, oysters, clams, lobster, salmon, dairy : fat free or reduced fat, skimmed milk, and yogurts.

Vegetables are baked potatoes with skin or other styles, preferably not fried, spinach, peas, lima beans, lentils, and dried beans of any color or kind. Grains are whole-wheat bread, cereal, and oatmeal products.

ASTHMA

Asthma is a paroxysmal dyspnea accompanied by wheezing caused by spasm of the bronchial tubes or by swelling of their mucous membrane. No age and nobody is exempt. But asthma usually occurs most frequently in childhood or early adulthood. People affected with this disease may assume a hunched forward position and attempt to get more air.

Other allergic disorders may coexist. Recurrence and severity of attacks is greatly influenced by secondary factors, by mental or physical fatigue, by exposure to fumes, by endocrine changes at various periods in life and by emotional situations. Status asthmaticus, a continuous asthmatic state, may last for hours or days.

Origin: Extrinsic Causes

The origin extrinsic causes are allergens inhaled in the air, pollen, mold spores, animal dander, dust or infection of the respiratory tract. Occasionally, foods like eggs, shellfish, chocolate, or drugs like aspirin may precipitate an attack. Extrinsic asthma is due to some environmental allergic factors.

Intrinsic Causes

In some cases, asthma develops in persons with allergies of unknown etiology. It may be precipitated by infection of the upper or lower respiratory tracts. Intrinsic asthma is assumed to be due to some endogenous cause because no external cause can be found.

Bronchial Asthma

Allergic asthma is a common form of asthma due to hypersensitivity to an allergen.

Cardiac Asthma

Asthma that is secondary to heart disease.

Intrinsic Asthma

Due to some endogenous cause because no external cause can be found.

Thymic Asthma

Asthma caused by sudden closure of the larynx that usually occurs in children and believed to result from enlargement of the thymus.

Almost Anything Can Promote Asthma

To my knowledge and some scientists, almost anything in life in general can promote an asthma attack. Sometimes you can get clues preceding an attack. Other times the attacks are sudden.

For example, change of seasons, temperatures, scents, fragrances, foods, ingredients in foods, cosmetics, exercises, leather, fur, animals, pets, people around you, pumping gas, heating system, fan, vent, noise, lights bright or dim, being upset, under pressure, stress, anxiety, other illness, smoke, wood burning, alcohol, bleach, Clorox, chlorine, chemicals, people, dust, mold, hair, dandruff, good or bad smell, snow, snowstorm, rain, cold, hot, warm temperature, heat, rain, shower or bath, brushing teeth, toothpaste, mouthwash, smell of ink in the printer from newspaper, stress from bills, wood-burning smoke, cigarette and cigar smoking, laughing hard, or crying, lovemaking, fighting, for woman having your menstruation, being pregnant, wearing condom, birth control pills, insect bites, pesticide, sprays, being sad or very happy, etc. You name it, can cause an asthma attack.

Sometimes some people with asthma history must be cautious at all times and carry an inhaler, make sure of a renewal at all times even if this person didn't have an asthma attack for ten to fifteen years. This person can certainly have an attack from an unforecasted snowstorm while out shopping for the holidays. Especially if this person happened to forget the inhaler at home in a different pocketbook, that is a sure asthma attack from change in temperature and anxiety.

Although some people can have a lot of allergens that can cause an allergic type of asthma attack, to my knowledge after over thirty years of research, experience, and experiment with all types of asthma, no one ever has all types of asthma and all allergens.

TREATMENT

Acute asthma may be relieved by a number of drugs such as epinephrine, ephedrine, cromolyn sodium, or aminophylline. For persistent asthma (status asthmaticus), the use of adrenaline adrenocortical hormones may be required. Although their use may provide dramatic relief, these hormones should be used only as long as necessary to control the acute asthmatic attack. Prolonged use of adrenocortical hormones will lead to development of serious side effects. The use of sedatives and expectorants is sometimes necessary. In all cases, efforts should be made to control causative factors including the component of the disease due to emotional disturbance, especially in the intrinsic group. Elimination of antigen or counteractivities such as immunization, desensitization, or hyposensitization is desirable for asthma due to infection of the respiratory tract, an antibiotic should be used to control infection or prevent recurrence.

Sometimes, some people with asthma must be cautious at all times and carry an inhaler and make sure of a renewal at all times also even if this person didn't have an attack for ten to fifteen years. Certainly, this person can have one attack from an unforecasted snowstorm. Especially if the person happens to forget their inhaler at home or in a different pocket or purse. Some good things with asthma are sometimes someone can have very bad asthma attacks for a long period in his or her life doing everything and taking every medication prescribed by a cohort of doctors without good result. But if by accident or serendipity, this person happens to move from his or her native land across the ocean to a new faraway land and society; he or she can get the best surprise in life, that "ta-daaaaaa!" No more asthma, no need for medication, and "Vive la belle vie" and do everything that he or she could not do before. But always be on guard, you never know! For some people, only a few things promote an asthma attack.

STATISTICS

Asthma is hard and common in any place people live and at any age. But for children in inner cities who were poor and young mothers giving birth to premature children without prenatal care, it's worse. The poorer is the community, the higher is the statistics for asthma for children who are forced to live in crowded buildings in some projects in unsanitary conditions faraway from health-care facilities. In these projects, people smoke, drink alcohol, and are in turmoil most of the time. Meanwhile, these premature children's lungs are not fully developed because human lungs of children born before full term do not have a substance called surfactant. This substance looks like cream cheese or sour cream that coats the lung tissue, making it pliable, soft, elastic, capable of folding for the inhale exhale for a perfect breathing process or respiration. In the United States, actually the statistics is 76,000,000 for all, and children count 90 percent of it.

Treatment and Prevention

Fortunately with proper medical and parental care, good nutrition, hygienic living conditions, and education about asthma, these children can lead a normal life and outgrow their childhood asthma.

For everyone with asthma, keep your surroundings or living area clean, with clean air, unpolluted, quiet, with sunlight through the windows in daytime and electrical soft light bulb at night. Keep your living area dry, free from dust, humidity, mold, smell of chemicals, fragrance, and bad or good smells.

Keep a diary of foods and activities. Keep a mild, quiet, and moderate atmosphere, never too hot, not too cold, but cool or warm. Don't be in a place that is too noisy or too quiet. Listen to soft classical music with a monotonous tone most of the time. Touching, cuddling, meditation, and imagery can prevent or slow down asthma attacks. Avoid heated arguments, discussions, screaming, yelling, confrontation, loud music, noisy crowds, irritating people and conditions. Don't be around complex, difficult, hardheaded, and too competitive people. Try to be around pleasant, courteous, generous, understanding, good, and nice positive people if you can find some in this world. Stay away from negative, hypercritical, and mean people.

Although you need to be sociable, it is better to be alone, not lonely, than to be around the type of people that can make you sick even if they are your loved ones. Do not be afraid to change jobs or place of residence if that compromises your health and promote bad asthma attacks.

Foods and Drinks

As far as foods and drinks, you are the boss, the doctor, the know-how with your diary. Eat any food of the five food groups that contain protein, enzymes, vitamins, and minerals that you are not allergic to. But stay away from animal fats, trans fats, a lot of sodium, a lot of sugar, artificial food and drinks, processed contaminated foods and drinks. Eat only fresh food cooked by you or that you know are cooked in a sanitary manner. Drink 100 percent fruit juice, spring water, low-fat dairy milk. Know how to read labels for nutritional and chemical contents. Stay at your ideal weight, not overweight, not too much underweight. Stay away from artificial, processed, contaminated, uncooked, acidic and alkali foods that you will find in my first book T.H.A.T.S. The Health Assistance to Some *to cover the type of food preparation, protection, and nutrition you should know to fight most diseases and lead a healthy life. Eat only foods that don't make you sick, according to your diary or observation and not what people tell you to eat.*

Remember, with asthma or many other diseases, you are the doctor, the nutritionist, the boss, the pharmacist, the cook, etc., and no one else. According to my observation, even children or toddlers stand up to their parents when it comes to their food intake. Some of them cry, say no, shake their heads, kick, scratch, and spit out the food or drink that their parents feed them and grab something else and eat or drink it and calm down. Their natural instinct dictates to them what is good or bad for their asthmatic condition without a diary that they can't keep yet.

Good Advice

With some diseases or conditions like asthma, for example, people with or who have had asthma should be almost always prepared in case he or she suddenly has an attack.

Although asthma is a chronic disease, some people can outgrow it, not have it for decades, but should never be unprepared.

To me, no matter how long you go without having an asthma attack, almost always have an inhaler in your purse, car, desk drawer at work, or bedroom dresser drawer. Make sure you check your inhaler for expiration dates and optimum quality for immediate operation. It can be prescription or an over-the-counter inhaler. If over-the-counter, check expiration date, color, function, and operation. If it is a prescription, ask your primary physician for a renewal. Do not change brand or ingredients. If you go to a new doctor, remember your prescription or write a list of your usual drugs.

The point that I am trying to make is that people can have a sudden asthma attack after two decades or more without an attack. Sometimes all it takes is a long cold winter, a bad allergy season, an epidemic of flu or other viruses, or being exposed to allergens such as the following:

Closet smokers
Closet alcoholics
Drug addicts
Too much fragrance
New chemicals being added to your food, toiletries, clothing, bedding material, and detergents

Fortunately, we have labels in almost everything. Therefore, take time to read them before buying because it can prevent a lot of misery.

BLOOD PRESSURE

Blood pressure, as popularly used, is the pressure determined indirectly, existing in the large arteries at the height of the pulse wave, the systolic intra-arterial pressure exerted by the blood vessel on the wall of any vessel. This pressure reaches the highest values in the left ventricle during systole. It decreases in the arterial creases and is lower in capillaries than in the arteries. The systolic arterial blood pressure rises during activity or excitement and falls during sleep. In the normal, relaxed, sitting adult, it may be as low as 100 and as high as 140 mm of mercury (4g). The following findings are considered abnormal: systolic pressure persistently above 140, diastolic persistently above 100, pulse pressure persistently greater than 50.

VARIATION

Blood pressure varies with age, sex, altitude, muscular development, according to states of worry, fatigue, and to race. Usually it is lower in women than men, in black than white, Caucasian, yellow Asiatic, and red or Indian. It is also lower in children and young adults and higher in elderly individuals.

DIASTOLE, HYPERTENSION, HYPOTENSION, PULSE PRESSURE, SYSTOLE

Blood pressure during the relaxation phase between heartbeats is normally about 80 mm. Hg is dependent primarily upon the elasticity of the arteries and peripheral resistance, which in turn is dependent upon caliber of arterioles and capillaries BP.

Direct measurement of determining the blood pressure in one of several arteries is done by placing a sterile needle or small catheter inside an artery and having the blood pressure transmitted through that system to a suitable recorder. As the blood pressure fluctuates, the changes are recorded graphically.

INDUCED MEASUREMENT

Induced measurement is a simple external method for measuring blood pressure.

PALPATORY METHOD

PALPATORY method is when the same arm, usually the right, should be used each time the pressure is measured. The arm should be raised to heart level if the patient is sitting or kept parallel to the body if the patient is recumbent. The examination could result in a higher blood pressure reading. Either a mercury gravity or aneroid-manometer type of blood pressure apparatus may be used. The blood compression cuff should be the width and length appropriate for the size of the subject's arm: narrow (2.5) to (6 cm.) The deflate cuff is placed evenly and snugly around the upper arm so that the lower edge is about one inch above the point of the brachial artery where the bell of the stethoscope will be applied. While feeling the radial pulse, inflate the cuff until the pressure is about 30 mm above the point where the radial pulse was no longer felt and deflate the cuff slowly and record, as accurately as possible, the pressure at which the pulse returns to the radial artery. Systolic blood pressure is determined by this method while diastolic pressure cannot be determined by this method.

EXAMPLE OF BLOOD PRESSURE

One twenty over eighty indicates systolic pressure of 120 and diastolic of 80. Normal blood pressure in a healthy young person is about 100 to 140 mm of mercury systolic and 60 to 90 mm diastolic. Loss of resilience in the vascular tree and physiological changes of age must be considered when levels above 140 mm are obtained in apparently healthy older persons. The systolic is the greatest force caused by the contraction of the ventricle of the heart.

MY ADVICE

If you have hypertension (high blood pressure), walking daily, even with a cane or walker, can help you. If you are rehabilitating from a stroke and you are able to walk with a cane or walker, walking will help you reach your goal faster than without it.

TRUE STORY

This is a true story about my husband who was in his late thirties. At that time, he worked far away from home and could come home on days off. He was sick and diagnosed with high blood pressure. He was taking medication for it. At dinnertime, he pulled out a small white tablet from a bottle and placed it in his mouth. I said, "What is this? Give it to me." I looked at the medication and the bottle, found out that it was for high blood pressure. I said to him, "How long have you been taking this?" He answered, "Since last week. The doctor gave it to me." I grabbed the bottle and emptied it in the garbage can. I placed him on a high-fiber, low-sodium diet of lean poultry, fish, fat-free dairy, fruits, vegetables, whole grain, beans, legumes along with eight eight-ounce glasses of spring water and a one-hour walk daily. At his next checkup before the renewal of his medication, which was after three months, his blood pressure was 110/70. The doctor called his staff members and told them. He couldn't believe it, and he asked two other doctors to check it too. The doctor said "You are a good patient! You took all your medication, and I am going to give you some more."

My husband said, "No, I only took three tablets. My wife emptied the bottle full of tablets in the garbage can, placed me on her own diet and exercise plan, and I feel fine." Since that time, he has never been sick or had to take any medication. My husband goes to the doctors for checkups and makes sure to tell me his test results before touching any drugs even a topical cream or ointment.

Another True History

A few years ago, my husband visited another doctor who told him that everything was fine, his blood pressure was excellent, and he was in good health. The doctor asked him what he did for such good health, and my husband answered, "My wife placed me on a diet and exercise program she created for me, and I feel great and love it!" The doctor replied, "You can eat whatever you want: fatty foods, salt, fast-food and you don't have to be on a diet all your life. I can give you some medications for that!" My husband said, "No thank you." He told me when he came home, "Honey, the doctor thinks that I am crazy enough to listen to him and eat all the bad foods I want and take medications from him for everything I want." We both laughed at the doctor. We continue to go for checkups and never touched one single pill or tablet and remained healthy up to now in 2013. These stories or examples for high blood pressure or hypertension are also in my first book T.H.A.T.S., The Health Assistance to Some.

VITAMIN D

According to an article I recently read, Vitamin D can lower blood pressure.

Taking vitamin D supplements can lower your blood pressure as effective as some drugs, researchers have discovered. In a blind study, volunteers with high blood pressure who took the real deal saw their high blood pressure lowered dramatically compared to those who took placebos. About 90 percent of the body's vitamin D supply comes from sunlight, and so many people suffer from low amount of the vitamin D. As per a paper presented to the European society, the volunteers who took seventy to eighty micrograms of vitamin D for five months also had a significant decrease in central blood pressure measurement close to the heart.

Vitamin D may not be a cure to high blood pressure, however; there is a possibility it may decrease a great deal. A good way to control high blood pressure without drugs and their nasty side effects is to take vitamin D as supplements. At your next annual visit to the doctor, ask him or her to test you for vitamin D.

Good news!!!! Some scientists have discovered that you can control and even cure your high blood pressure without expensive and risky drugs. What it takes for most people is a few lifestyle changes: just try hard to lose some excess pounds and you will see a decrease in your systolic or top number and diastolic or bottom number from 1 to 2 (mm) millimeter on the testing instrument in your doctor's office during your next visit. For any laypeople, it does not seem to be much, but for people in the medical profession, it's colossal!!! Better yet, eliminating just half of a teaspoon of salt in your daily intake or diet will reduce your systolic and diastolic pressure by 6 to 5 and 3 to 2 mm. By increasing fruits and vegetables in your diet, you will drop more weights and decrease of 10 to 12 points in your systolic pressure and 5 to 3 points in your diastolic reading.

DIET FOOD INTAKE

Diet or food intake to prevent, decrease, and cure high blood pressure include all food containing calcium, potassium but low in fat such as milk, yogurt, cheese, ice cream, etc., because they contain calcium. Calcium can help keep blood vessel walls' muscle tissue supple so that they can operate efficiently. Bananas also help with blood pressure problems because they contain potassium. Other food that can help in controlling blood pressure problems are salmon, spinach, sweet potato, walnut, seafood, for example, crab, lobster, oysters, and eggs specially the white part. All the above foods can help in controlling, decreasing, and disappearing all blood pressure problems for good. If you are a big fan of salad, make a big bowl of green salad that include romaine lettuce, watercress, and all the green leafy vegetables and salad you know. Next sprinkle olive oil, roasted garlic, dices of yellow, white, and purple onion on top of it to have a ball by eating a bowl daily!!!!

Another good food to control high blood pressure without drugs (too good to be true!!!) is the potato, the white one. The potato is not just a bad starchy food full of calories that make you fat, raise your blood sugar level, your fatty cholesterol, and your blood pressure. On the contrary, potato is a nutritional powerhouse food to have a spectacular place in your diet! A regular potato contains 160 calories only and no fat, no cholesterol, and no refined sugar. Potato contains very little carbohydrates, lots of vitamin C, iron, potassium, and protein compared to broccoli, spinach, and many other vegetables that people prefer to eat. If you wash it well, cook it with the skin, and eat it without peeling, you will get all the benefit including a large amount of fiber also. Please control your blood pressure with good eating habits, activities, normal weight, eight glasses of spring water in twenty-four hours, two to three cups of tea, any color or type, such as decaffeinated or not, and a good night's sleep, that will be next, and you will be back to normal very soon.

SLEEP

According to me and some other scientists, sleep is very important in controlling almost every type of diseases and conditions people can have. Therefore, everybody should try to have a good night's sleep every night. It means seven to nine hours with minor interruption, according to me and other doctors or scientists. But to me, the normal time is eight hours of sleep just like I believe that the number eight (8) is a magic number in our life. I tell you why. The number of water to drink in 24 hours is eight glasses of eight ounces. In the medical profession, if a patient can count to ten but skip the number 8 each time or only once, the patient is having a stroke; in the Catholic religion, children have first communion at eight years old; most jobs or employments people work eight hours per shift or day. To confirm my argument about sleep importance, I have included this article that I had read not too long ago.

INSOMNIA LEADS TO HYPERTENSION

Insufficient sleep shows as a major risk factor in hypertension, according to a research study conducted at Columbia University School of Public Health. They discovered that men and women who routinely get five hours or fewer hours of sleep a night are 60 percent more likely to suffer from hypertension, chronic high blood pressure that can lead to irreversible heart disease and stroke. "In people deprived of sleep, the average work done by the heart increases, and can lead to irreversible changes in the heart and blood vessels," says coauthor Dr. Dolores Malaspina.

CANCER

Long ago, the word "cancer" as a disease was almost taboo, too scary to talk about and even painful to say for some people sensitive as me. For example, I love people so much that even in television commercials, if it is something very painful like the advertisement to stop smoking, I always run away if I can't turn off the TV because someone else is watching with me. Right now, writing about it makes tears drip to my chest. For years, I have been procrastinating about writing this subject name "Cancer."

I started collecting information about this disease since anyone can count on their fingers how many cases were known of this disease in this country. My documentation is so vast that I had to get rid of some materials once in a while. I remember the first case known to me since I was a curious child listening to adult conversation. I was about five to six years old. I also remember the name of the person, followed up of the conversation.

TECHNOLOGY

To me, technology is a double-edged saw that gives and cures, the same way most of us enjoy technology, the same way we have to agree that it is the main part of this disease "cancer." To make a perfect equation, let us say the same way some technologies give cancer and some other diseases. It is the same way technology cures cancer and other diseases.

According to my observation, survey, and documentation, the younger people in recent time compared to old-timers or older people have more cases of cancer. The richer people who can afford a lot of commodities, luxury, and technological trinkets that money can buy have more cases of cancer. Although for some diseases including cancer, old age is a factor, to me it is not in this century. Again according to my observation and documentation, the old and poor who can't afford most of technological stuffs, have less cases of cancer than the rich and famous and young who only know and use one *way in life, which is more and more technology, are the ones having more and more cancers. Sometimes you may find some older people who lived a not too healthy lifestyle in their youth have cancer later on. Nevertheless, the majority of people with cancer are in our century.*

Not too long ago, people used to have one case of cancer that if metastasized moved to another spot or part of the body. But at present, people can have several different cancers in many places or organs at the same time. Some people can have brain cancer treated and after fifteen years have another cancer in the colon treated for two years and have another one for one year and die from it. I would not believe it if that was not a case of a close relative. This is a case that I followed for seventeen years. I will come back to it and report it in great detail.

AN EXAMPLE OF TECHNOLOGY

For example, some of us old-timers can remember when all telephones had a cord attached to the wall beside the electrical cord. Next we had a little wireless portable trinket that we carried in our pockets or belts for men and for women in pocketbooks or purses. It was incredible for almost everyone, especially for people in the medical profession. If one of the doctors, nurses, and other laboratory and X-ray technicians are deep down in a subbasement, they can hear the beeps, look at the numbers, recognize the name of the caller, and go to a fixed-to-the-wall telephone, and last, call back the person who beeped. Again, this invention goes back to technology. And most technologies we benefit from at present are from the space program with all the radiations from the solar system. I KNEW IT WAS GOING TO BE A PAYBACK. I DIDN'T KNOW HOW AND WITH WHAT DISEASE. Therefore, I started my work as soon as possible. What I knew for sure is that behind any invention there is a coin. And in any "coin," there are two sides. As you can see in my book named T.H.A.T.S., I referred to some inventions my son and I made by curiosity to pass time; we destroyed them right away and ripped up the written materials to shred. Both of us know that these trinkets can be useful, bring a lot of money, but can be detrimental to our health also.

Let's go back to telephones as part of technology. From fixed by a wire on the wall to beepers, next to cordless phones, next to cell phones, now you can use cell phones as a computer to text, e- mail, send messages, go online, browse the Internet, take pictures, send them all over the world, have friends, news from all over the world, watch television, movies, etc. In the medical profession, there are zillions of new technologies that people are using every day and night, 24-7, from Monday to Sunday, and January to December.

DOUBLE-EDGE SAW

The double-edge saw is in the entertainment, media, movies, flashes, lights, cameras, the rich and famous. For example, in some commercials, with a short sentence, you can have a person repeat the same sentence for twelve takes, which means that individuals must have a camera flash that lights twelve times over this person before that individual can hope to have the part and make the money that comes with it. Another example of a person I knew and loved as a relative who worked in the medical profession as an X-ray technician for forty years. For over thirty years, he worked eight hours a day in two reputable hospitals close to each other, making sixteen hours a day per week. I am not surprised of what happened to him after he retired.

CASE STUDY OR HISTORY

One day, this person started having headaches and took over-the-counter medications and used cold compresses. But the headache continued. He went to see a doctor, had a battery of tests, and was diagnosed with brain cancer stage 2. He had surgery to remove the cancerous tumor. After a few months had passed, he felt fine, had his checkup, returned to work, and the headaches came back. The same patient returned to the same doctor again for more tests and found out that the doctor had left a major part of the tumor inside of his head. He had surgery again to remove the rest of the cancerous tumor and had more chemotherapy again and was finally cured from brain cancer. The patient went back to work and stayed free of cancer for fifteen years. This was the doctor's mistake.

The patient, Mr. A, as a knowledgeable, educated, and a careful gentlemen, continued to go for annual checkups with great results except this time. The doctor found something abnormal in his abdomen. The doctor sent him for a battery of tests. Guest what? The result was colon cancer. Three years later, after being treated, he retired, enjoying life with his beautiful wife and his son, done with getting up to the alarm clock, living in a small apartment near the workplace far away from his family, isolated from relatives and friends. He said, "That's it. I can finally be happy this time in the warm climate of Florida, wearing cargo shorts, give parties, go to the beach," which were all he needed before he died.

Unfortunately, while bathing in the sun, his wife noticed that his feet were swelling. Since he had no pain, he never noticed that. The next day, he started soaking them in warm and cold water thinking that it is because he went jogging the day before. Meanwhile the swelling continued and came and went by closer intervals. Now came the time to go to the doctor. His wife reminded him, "Honey, don't forget to call and make an appointment with the doctor for your feet." After a battery of tests as usual, he found out that it was liver cancer stage 3. He started treatment again, but this time he died rapidly. It was too late. It is possible that this time his cancer in the colon had metastasized to the liver.

CANCER

BENIGN MALIGNANT NEOPLASIA

To talk about cancer, let us start with the cells in animals, men and women, and the cells themselves. One of the things that we have to be concerned with is the life cycle of cells. About 4 million of cells divide every second. Three hundred fifty billion divide in a day. Every single time a cell passes in a phase of the cycle, there is a risk of having cancer. Every time a cell divides, malignant neoplasm of 100 different diseases happen as cancers, such as in the lungs in men, in the breasts in women, also the rest of different types of cancers that we all know by now.

What makes someone develop cancer are the following:

Age
Abnormal growth
Neoplasm, which are new abnormal cells
Tumors
Aberrant cell growth
Malignant cells
Neoplasia, which is new growth that is abnormal

TUMOR

ABERANT CELLULAR GROWTH CANCER

CANCER is malignant growth that includes three specific varieties:

1. Abnormal cell division
2. Invasion of normal tissue
3. Spread to distant host cell differentiation (transformation how cells function live determine the above and plus how cells behave)

What happens to malignant cells at the cellular level?

AT cellular level, which comprises cancer, a group of diseases of cells develop at abnormal cellular growth with lack of control at cell level. Again, at cellular level, some cells contain certain components of the cells, which are diseased.

MOLECULAR WIZE

Molecular wiz abnormality, cancer is a group division caused by abnormal molecules in the nucleus. While in the nucleus, cancer is a group of diseases caused by three basic broad subgroups of cancers.

These cancers group are as follows:

1. Carcinoma
2. Sarcoma
3. Leukemia/lymphoma

CARCINOMA

Carcinoma Group

Carcinoma group is a group of abnormal cells in the epithelial origin invading surrounding tissue that spread within the host connective tissue, sarcoma/carcinoma, and fibrous tissue also.

LYNPHOID/LEUKEMIA

This is blood-forming cells in bone marrow lymph node that invade the mononuclear phagocytic system and other structures.

NEOPLASM CLASSIFICATION

The neoplasm classification is done according to two variables, which are the following:

1. *Malignant*
2. *Benign*

NEOPLASM CLASSIFICATION

According to this classification, some cells can be part of cell origin.

SQUAMOS/BASAL

This category include papilloma, carcinoma gland epithelium. The B group includes polyp or adenoma, myocitic granulocytic (leukemia)

ANOTHER THEM TERATE = MONSTER

Teratemo is a monstrous-sized tumor in the testicular area, which people having it does poorly

Testicular = teratocarcinoma or a benign form of teratoma

STAGES OF NEOPLASM

The stages of neoplasm describes the extent of disease in any given point.

T - O stage = Tumor is not bad
M - O = No need for chemo, cancer had just started
T4 M4 N4 = too far, is gone

THE REASON TO DETERMINE SURVIVAL RATE

The stage classification has three different reasons:

1. *to determine survival rate*
2. *using norm to facilitate exchange between agencies or medical centers*
3. *to determine related merit of different methods of treatment*

UNIVERSAL CLASSIC is T N M/T M N

This provides general principles of stages that in turn provide normal standards for stages

T = tumor/ primary lesion and extent
M = distant metastasis
N = Lymph node
T I S
T = 1 to 4, which indicate ascending degree of tumor size of which 4 is pretty far gone or last stage. It goes from 1 to 4 and with 0 as having no cancer.
M X = Amount and extent of metastasis and can't be assessed.

Prostatic cancer metastasizes to bone and breast cancer too. Both types need bone scan done very often.

STAGES

Stage 1 (T I No MO) = limited to organ of origin lesion operable and no node no spread; 70 to 90 percent chance of survival.
Stage 2 (T II N I MO) = first station lymph node environment; although complete tumor has begun to spread, there is 45 to 55 percent of survival.
Stage 3 (T3 N2 MO) = The mass is extensive, some invasion to bone area; lesion is operable, may be acceptable to certain amount of the disease remain chance is 15 to 25 percent.
Stage 4 (T4 N3 MI TMX) = evidence of distance metastasis beyond survival lesion operable chance O–5 percent chance.

Difference between benign and malignant:

BENIGN NEO

1. Retain cells that are of similar structure to cells from which they derive.
2. They are much more cohesive than malignant cells.
3. They grow evenly from the center of the neoplasm.
4. They have well-defined border edges.
5. They are usually encapsulated cells that typical push surrounding tissue away.
6. Growth is slower and limited to one area.
7. Blood supply is less profuse and there is less chance of recurrence; recurrence rarely necrosis.

MAGLIGNANT

1. Malignant cells are cells with abnormal nucleus.
2. These cells have abnormal chromosomes.
3. These cells don't look like cells of origin.
4. These cells are not cohesive.
5. These cells have irregular patterns.
6. These cells have no capsule they invade, take over surrounding tissue.
7. These cells have the ability to metastasize after surgical intervention.
8. These cells cause systemic problems, such as bone defect, coagulation, clotting, mobilized mental status, and chemical change.

NEOPLASM THEORY OF CAUSATION

None of the theories are for sure and there are four different proposed theories.

1. Somatic mutation
2. Aberrant differentiation
3. Virus activation
4. Cell selection

Somatic mutation was formulated by Bauer in early 1928. He says that certain abnormality within the genes is "mutational changes," induced by carcinogenic agent A or B, or hereditary susceptibility. Abnormality within chromosomes has Trisomie Down Syndrome, higher incidence of Leukemia, Chronic Malicitic, Philadelphia chromosome, translocation of chromosome 22.

Neurofibromatosis is a severe form of cancer, "café aux lait" skin cancer. Epigenetic theory, an aberrant differentiation theory, states that neoplastic change may result from disturbances in regularity of normal genes due to some type of repression in adult differentiated tissue. Other reasons are turning on and off the normally (doing) inactivated genes. There is some type of alteration in the embryonic growth and development in activation or repression; if yes everyone is susceptible to cancer in that case or theory.

VIRUS ACTIVATION: Oncogenic virus is linked to neoplasm genome to certain infected cells, which will alter the offspring or progeny and genetic makeup, so the host does not contract the cancer, but the offspring does. DNA virus is actually incorporated into the genes of the host type C virus, "ongenic virus," causing leukemia. Type B RNA virus is associated with breast cancer.

DNA EPSTEIN-BARR VIRUS causes a certain type of leukemia, mononuclear DNA type of virus associated with herpes type nasopharyngeal. BURKITT'S LYMPHOMA somewhere in Africa is another type of cancer. Cell selection, in which neoplasm develop in sequential pattern due to certain substances although not carcinogenic themselves, can promote carcinogenic growth. This theory is linked to an immunodeficiency individual with this type of cancer.

Some types of carcinogen:

1. *carbon monoxide*
2. *fumes from car*
3. *physical carcinogen*
4. *polyciclicaromatic hydrocarbons found in tobacco smoke*
5. *auto exhaust*
6. *product of combustion, the above cause: lips, tongue, laryngeal, lung, nasopharyngeal cancers.*

When exposed to aromatic amines, benzene, pesticides, spray, insecticide chemical, certain foods we eat, mothballs all are potent carcinogenic agents. Other carcinogenic agents are insect repellent, which is linked to bladder cancer. Rat roaches poison primarily certain chemo drugs, all metatrexcide, nitrogen, food nitrate, ham, bacon, pickles, pastrami, corned beef, certain natural products such as aspergillis flavus color in meat, barley, corn, peas, rice, some fruits, and almost all nuts are linked to liver cancer.

Meat is very potent, especially red meat; the color red makes cows fat. Meat cooked rare especially gives cancer. It is better to cook all meat longer. Other potent cancer-causing agents that give bladder cancer are antifungal agents, jock itch under the toes, tinactin, macatin. Other potent agents for bladder and reproductive organ cancers are asbestos, nickel, ultraviolet rays, radiation, and diethanol.

CARCINOGEN AGENTS OR FACTORS:

Smoking, sunbathing, drinking alcohol, and eating raw fish all give stomach cancer. This type of cancer is higher in the Japanese because of their diet with a lot of raw fish. A lot of types of cancers have to do with individual diet depending on what consists the diet, such as high cholesterol, fat, higher fiber, which is good, and lower fiber and more fat, which is bad.

MULTIPLE SEX PARTNERS

Sex and multiple partners at a young age can cause cervical cancer. Uncircumcised partners can cause cancer.

NO CHILDREN

Women with no children are prone to breast cancer as well as women who never get pregnant, begin early and end late menarche and started early or late menopause.

THEORY LINKING HORMONE TO CANCER

Increased hormone levels at certain times can make an individual prone to neoplasm.

INFECTUOS PROCESSES

Nutrition
Drug therapy
Insect control
Cleanliness
Hand washing
Bacteria
Viruses
Worm
Microbial agent has mutant strain that are resistant to antibiotic.

For me, people should have a positive attitude and start everything early as possible. Also, people should investigate, compare, listen to others with knowledge and pay attention to what they feel, hear, see, eat, smell, taste, and touch; and if in doubt of anything, talk to someone about it before it develops too much and becomes too late. Just remember that you don't have to be a scientist. All you need is to pay attention, be yourself, and share with someone else such as a good friend, a family member, your primary doctor that can advise you on how to start with your care as early as possible. My advice to people in doubt of any disease is to have a doctor that you can trust, whom you know for a long time, who has become like a family member or a good friend. It should be a person who can listen to you, give you a special time to look, touch, listen, and consult with you.

BREAST CANCER

Three Ways to Beat Breast Cancer

Mammogram: The American College of Obstetricians and Gynecologists recommends having a mammogram at age forty and then at least every two years for women older than age fifty.

According to an article I read in 2009, researchers at the American Institute recently reviewed 954 clinical studies and concluded that a few simple and easy lifestyle changes can reduce women's risk of getting breast cancer by 40 percent. That means 70,000 fewer women will be diagnosed each year. Specifically, there are three steps you can take today that experts feel represent the best ways to protect yourself.

First of all, strive to get your weight within normal limits; women with low body fat are less likely to develop postmenopausal breast cancer. Body fat plays a role in the production of certain hormones and proteins that encourage tumor in the breast tissue.

Second, try to get at least thirty minutes of exercise on most days. Physical activities decrease the level of estrogen and androgen that are associated with breast cancer.

Exercise will also help you to maintain a healthy weight and provide your body's cells with adequate amounts of oxygen. Your workout doesn't have to be at a formal exercise station. It can consist of brisk walking, vigorous housework or gardening, anything that increases breathing and raises your heart rate.

Third, limit your alcohol consumption. One study found that five drinks a week will increase your breast cancer risk by 5 percent. When alcohol is digested, it releases cancer-causing chemicals into the body. "Booze" also boosts breast cancer risk by upping estrogen levels.

In addition to these three steps, younger women can benefit by breast-feeding. Research shows a 3 percent drop in breast cancer risk for every five months spent nursing. Breast-feeding limits the production of cancer-causing hormones. It also promotes the rapid turnover of breast cancer cells, eliminating those with DNA that are susceptible to malignant mutation.

Statistics for Breast Cancer

An estimated 182,500 women in the USA alone will be diagnosed with breast cancer, and approximately 41,000 women will die of the disease. That was in 2008.

What promotes or increase this number?

Drugs: Like hormones for women after menopause, for example, estrogen and progestin.

Age: Women sixty years old and older.

Race: Whites, except Hispanics.

Hereditary: If your mother, sister, or daughters have it.

Genetics: BRCA 1 and BRCA 2 from your test.

Weight: If you are obese or overweight, close to and past menopausal age, keep your weight five pounds less or over, never more than twenty-two pounds over or under. Women over or under by that much should do their best to increase or decrease that weight according to their normal weight, using BMI scale.

Menstrual periods: People who started to menstruate early, such as before the age of twelve and stop after fifty-five, which is more than the regular period.

Age to give birth: Giving birth after thirty to first child or never giving birth.

Breast tissue: Dense or fatty breast or density tissue on your mammogram test results.

Abnormal breast cells found in biopsy: Abnormal or atypical hyperplasia or lobular carcinoma.

Cancer statistics in 2014 are climbing by the minute due to counterfeits with deadly chemical cancer-causing poisonous materials in almost all of our popular brands of cosmetics, toiletries, and clothing accessories.

New Test Predicts Breast Cancer Risk

Researchers have developed the world's first test to accurately predict the risk of breast cancer in individual women. This is a crucial advance because the current testing method called Gail Model can only determine the average risk among a large group of women. When it comes to individuals, it's littler than a blind guess. The new test counts the number of acini, small milk-producing structures in breast lobules. The more acini and the bigger the lobules, the greater a woman's chances of getting breast cancer. Lobules normally decrease in number as a woman ages, eventually disappearing entirely; but if a woman aged fifty-five still has a significant number present, her risk of breast cancer triples. Lynn Hartmann, a cancer specialist who led the research team, advises doctors to use the test in conjunction with family history and genetic testing to gain an even more accurate prediction.

General Knowledge about Cancer

For women

Colonoscopy: Colon cancer kills more women than ovarian, uterine, and cervical cancer combined. Suggested screening is the same as for men.

Pap test: This test can detect cervical cancer in its earliest most curable stages. Experts say if Pap smears have been normal for years, then test every thirty-six months.

Mammogram: The American College of Obstetrician and Gynecologists recommends having a mammogram at age forty and then at least every two years for women older than age fifty.

For men

PSA: The specific antigen test helps detect prostate cancer, which affects 1 in 6 men and is the second leading death cause in guys. Experts suggest screening every two years for ages fifty-five to sixty-nine.

Colonoscopy: Colon cancer is the third most common cancer in men and can be deadly. Start screening at age fifty and continue every ten years. Those with a family history of the disease should be tested more frequently as their doctor recommends.

The above is according to a recent report by Lynn Allison

COLON CANCER

Smoking and drinking raises the risk of colon cancer. George Institute for International Health: people who knock back more than seven drinks a week have a 60 percent greater chance of developing colorectal cancer than nondrinkers, a new study reveals. Obesity, diabetes, and eating red meats too often can also make you more vulnerable to the disease. In the same study, researchers found that moderate exercise reduces the risk slightly, but not enough to offset the consequences of unhealthy lifestyle habits.

According to new guidelines for colon exam, scientists at Mayo Clinic say a colonoscopy is a crucial test for the early detection of colon cancer, but many patients find it unpleasant and tend to avoid it. The problem is mad worse because approximately 15 percent of the test fail and have to be repeated due to faulty preparation. The usual prep involves switching to a diet of clear liquids forty-eight hours before the test. Doing so substantially improves the quality of the preparation. Doctors recommend liquids that contain plenty of electrolytes, such as broth and sports drinks.

LIVER Problem (CANCER)

Symptoms: diarrhea, midstomach pains, light (yellow, amber) or to dark (dark brown, black) stool.
Causes: Candy, beef, alcohol, medications, fat, toxin in air pollution, chemicals, garbage trucks. Toxic-clogged liver feels sluggish and will not do its job properly. Fatty foods such as fried chicken, butter, and lard will cause problems. A toxic-clogged liver can detoxify itself. It can even grow back and regenerate itself; this property is what makes liver transplants possible.

Below are foods you can use before running to your doctor:

Dandelion
Romaine lettuce
Arugula
Spinach
Probiotic yogurt (to prepare your own intestinal bacteria so that they benefit you)

Mix the following ingredients and drink it in the morning:

1/4 cup of warm water
Wedge of lemon (not lime)
A teaspoon of hot sauce

Commonly used foods:

Honey
Whole grain
Bananas
Yogurt
Garlic
Onion
Cooked grain (rice)
Whole-wheat barley
Oatmeal
Corn
Almost all vegetables

ORAL CANCER

An American dies of oral cancer every minute of every day, yet it is one of the easiest malignancies to treat if it is caught early enough. A new device allows your dentist to find the deadly disease before it progresses to the stage where it becomes difficult to treat. It's called Vizilite Plus and it's painless and quick. All you do is rinse your mouth with a cleansing solution then the dentist will shine Vizilite onto the tissue. Oral cancer is on the rise, and medical experts advise a routine exam, especially if you are older than forty, a smoker, and have red or white patches on your tongue or on the inside of your mouth.

Prevention

Eat foods high in vitamin C, green leafy vegetables, seafood and poultry, non-fatty foods (fried, excessive butter).
Use less white bleached flours and grains.
Eat less sugary foods.

Use baking soda and water solution as a mouth rinse.

THYROID CANCER

The following are good techniques for everyone, especially women, because more women are afflicted with thyroid cancer or thyroid diseases and problems than men:

Use a thermometer in the morning to check temperature: it should be between ninety-eight to ninety-nine degrees. If it is lower than ninety-eight degrees, investigate thyroid further; It may be hypothyroid. Use three fingers at the base of the throat just above the clavicle bone and beneath the Adam's apple. If you can feel the gland, it's a bad problem. Seek a professional medical evaluation for test.

If the thyroid is not working properly, you will age prematurely and it will not convert fat into energy, resulting in sluggish, lethargic, exhausted behavior and gaining weight. This disease is almost impossible to diagnose.

If you are suffering from hypothyroid, you need Iodine from salt; mushrooms, which are rich in a compound called selenium; and brazil nuts because they are rich in selenium also.

On the contrary, hyperthyroid can cause hyperactivity, resulting in rapid weight loss and dehydration.

If you suffer from hyperthyroid, drink plenty of water, try to rest by sitting down and reading, eat a snack, and take naps during the day.

The best help is to learn how to conserve energy.

CANCER-CAUSING ACTIVITIES AND THEIR REMEDIES

Smoking	Quitting
Overeating	Moderation
Drinking	Being sober

Procrastination	Motivation/energizing
Sitting Down	Exercising

CANCER-FIGHTING FOODS

Collard Greens	Interrupt blood supply to the tumor
Beans	Full of fiber
Tomato (sweet tomato)	Antioxidant
Coffee	Polyphenol antioxidant (maximum of three cups a day)

Example Breakfast: 100-calorie breakfast consisting of nuts, protein, fruit, cereal, yogurt with or without fruit, oatmeal, and peanut butter (old-fashioned).

CHOLESTEROL

Cholesterol is a monohydric alcohol, a sterol widely distributed in animal tissue and occurring in the yolk of eggs, various oils, fats, nerve tissue of the brain and spinal cord, the liver, kidneys, and the adrenal glands. It can be synthesized in the liver and a normal constituent of bile. It is the principal constituent of most gallstones. It is important in metabolism, serving as a precursor of various steroid hormones, for example, sex hormones, adrenal corticoids.

Cholesterol Condition Types

There is a condition named cholesteroluria, which is the presence of cholesterol in urine.

There are two main cholesterols: the LDL or the fatty cholesterol and the HDL, the good cholesterol. To be healthy, we need to decrease the fatty cholesterol and increase the good cholesterol to give us the most, a total of 200 maximum and still be good or normal. If the reading is even 210 to 220, the reading is fair or close to borderline abnormal. Just know that in medicine, there is no completely good reading all the time because *medicine is not an exact, definite, final, and permanent science. Medicine deals with parameter, progressive, changeable, active, mobile, unrealistic, controllable or uncontrollable, unknown to us, which we call miracle sometimes because we don't really know the disease or condition yet. Even with all the tests, machines, and technology, we are still in the dark most of the time. Therefore, at the present time, let us leave it as is.*

Example: A few years ago, we know that egg yolk or the yellow part of an egg was the cause of cholesterol and we should not eat it. At present, some scientists say that the egg's yolk or the yellow part of the eggs can be eaten without fear of cholesterol rise. It was a mistake, according to the same scientists. What I always believe in was eating everything in moderation. To me, if egg yolks were the cause of the fatty LDL cholesterol, some nations would have only a few people left because their people ate egg yolks in everything and every day. These people put eggs in meat loaf, meatballs, pies, crepes, mousse, sauces, breads, pancakes, rice and vegetables, soufflés, biscuits, cakes, etc. For some time up to now, a lot of people have been eating egg whites only and products made without egg yolk, which is great for their health.

According to my researches, experiments, and experience, I always know that it is animal fat that raises the fatty LDL cholesterol and decreases the good HDL cholesterol. Vegetable fats, fruits, and grains increase good cholesterol HDL and decrease fatty cholesterol LDL. With this knowledge, when you have your lab work done for annual checkup, ask your doctor to give you a copy of your lab report and interpret or find out what to do or eat according to the results with the information you read in this chapter. Once you understand the result, you can adjust it to a normal parameter with foods, exercises, and good habits. If you are not in the medical field and not sure about what you read above, ask your doctor about your test result and what that means and what can you do to make it right before you accept and take any medication or drugs. Don't forget to ask for alternatives, such as diet and activities.

FOODS TO EAT TO RAISE HDL GOOD CHOLESTEROL

To raise HDL or the good cholesterol, eat grains, whole grains; whole wheat; corn; brown rice or any color (less of the white); beans, dry or fresh, black, red, white, navy; garbanzo; or chickpeas, any way you want except raw or cooked with animal fats. Boil or soak or refrigerate overnight to decrease gas. Make chili with or without ground meat and tofu, cook with rice, cornmeal, millet, barley, or any whole grain you like. Make puree, soup, sauce, pie, salad, hot or cold, with beans.

NUTS: All nuts can decrease LDL or fatty cholesterol and increase HDL or good cholesterol. With cashew, brazil, chestnut, hazelnut, macadamia, pecan, peanut, peanut butter, make butter, oil, sauce, pie salad, candy, oil, salad, muffin, cake, ice cream, main dish, combo with vegetable, snack or a handful of nuts can increase HDL and decrease LDL.

SEEDS can increase HDL and decrease LDL. Use flaxseed, sunflower seeds, other good seeds and their oil can increase good HDL cholesterol and decrease LDL.

VEGETABLES: All vegetables, especially the green leafy vegetables and legumes can do a good job with increasing good cholesterol and decreasing bad cholesterol.

FRUITS: All fruits are good, and the best are avocado, grapefruits, lemons; and the rest of them, such as tomato, papaya, apple, pear, oranges, grapes, and bananas are good for cholesterol. Vegetables and fruits, cooked or raw, and green leafy salads are even better to prevent, decrease, or cure cholesterol problems.

WHAT TO AVOID: Animal fat, coconut and palm oil. Decrease or use moderately dairy products, such as eggs with yellow or yolk, milk, and yogurt. Other animal products should be fat free, skimmed or reduced fat, low fat. No butter, shortening, lard, etc. Eat and drink skimmed milk, fat-free margarine, or plant sterol. To remove the fat from your poultry, after seasoning, boil it for a few minutes; keep the juice for sauce or gravy. Next, bake, stir-fry or broil your poultry. Let the juice in the refrigerator cool off and look on top of it for the fat. Then next remove the fat collection with a spoon and throw it in the garbage before you eat it with your food.

CONDIMENT: Relish Indian, sweet, or any brand and kind that you like, salsa with onions, tomato, garlic, all kinds of mustard, a teaspoon daily in your food cooked or raw, olive oil, red, purple, yellow, white or green peppers and all other colors, tomato raw in salad, guacamole, or avocado salad, celery, lemonade, or little lemon juice and or a capful of vinegar on your salad or vinaigrette with red wine, apple cider, or white vinegar, a teaspoonful of honey in a full glass of warm water to drink before breakfast can make all cholesterol problems something of the past for you. So you never have to touch a pill with side effects from a bottle again. Continue to see your doctor for tests, annual checkups to make sure that your cholesterol is controlled.

If you really have an emergency that even the statin drugs would take too long to save your life, there is a new machine or device called the Liposorber that can literally flush the fatty cholesterol LDL out of your bloodstream in minutes the same way dialysis removes toxin from the blood of the kidney patients. But according to new research, you better not flush all your LDL or fatty cholesterol because like I always say, you need the bad cholesterol for your brain and your good health and also if the LDL and the foods that some scientists claimed were so bad, some people in some countries would have been very unhealthy.

In some tests at the University of North Carolina, the results have been like miracles. A level of fatty cholesterol LDL goes from 300 to 60 in just one session, according to Dr. Ross Simpson, head of the school of lipid clinic. According to statistics since 2010, heart disease is the leading cause of premature death among American men and women, and the leading cause of heart disease is cholesterol. Therefore, decrease or improve your cholesterol and prevent heart diseases, live healthier, and longer. Not so fast, according to new research of 2013, the bad cholesterol does not cause heart attack at all. The people with the bad cholesterol may have other problems, and together, that causes their heart attack. If the people have no other problems and only high bad cholesterol, these people can live healthy for a long time (Channel 5 Fox 5 TV in New York report, April 2013).

RED MEAT STEAK

By the way, for years, some scientists have been telling people to eliminate juicy steaks and burgers from their diet to reduce the risk of high fatty cholesterol LDL and prevent heart attack. Due to this belief, a majority of people cut out completely all red meats in their diet. They only eat fish, seafood, and chicken, which can reduce their level of red blood cells and cause anemia, iron, and other minerals, electrolytes and some vitamins deficiency. For this reason, you can't cut read meat completely from your diet. What you can do are choose your red meat carefully, buy good brand names that are organic, low-percent fat, taking your time to read labels or contents and eat your juicy burger with a bowl of green salad, whole-wheat bun, or a piece of juicy steak that you cook yourself at least once a month. And forget about fatty cholesterol LDL that scientists say is no longer bad for you and don't cause heart attacks anymore, which I always knew. Because if red meat had caused bad cholesterol that give heart attacks, there wouldn't be one French man alive by now. A piece of bloody juicy steak is their preferred food. And whole egg whites and yolks are their daily food in every meal. LDL cholesterol is just fat that our brain needs as lubricant to survive. This information is according to Fox Channel 5 New York City. Our scientists better look for something else in your diet that causes the diseases and heart attacks.

DIABETES

Definition of diabetes: In Greek, "diabetes" means "passing through," which is a general term for diseases characterized by excessive urination usually referred to as diabetes mellitus.

Diabetes brittle is an unpredictable variation in a person's glucose tolerance. This type of diabetes is particularly proved to be present in individuals whose diabetes developed during childhood.

Diabetes bronze is a disease of iron metabolism characterized by enlargement of the liver, pigmentation of the skin so that it takes a bronzed blue hue, diabetes mellitus, and frequently cardiac failure. It is a rare condition seen ten times as frequently in males as females. The majority of cases develop after forty years of age, which is also called hemochromatosis.

Diabetes chemical is a stage of diabetes mellitus in which the various tests for altered glucose metabolism other than fasting blood glucose level are abnormal, but there are no obvious clinical signs or symptoms of diabetes.

Diabetes endocrine is the diabetes mellitus associated with certain diseases of the pituitary, thyroid, or adrenal glands.

Diabetes Iatrogenic is the diabetes mellitus brought on by administration of drugs, such as corticosteroids, certain diuretics, or birth control pills.

Diabetes insipidus is the form when polyuria and polydipsia are caused by inadequate secretion of vasopressin, the antidiuretic hormone, by the neurohypophysis, which is the main portion of the posterior lobe of the pituitary gland. This form of diabetes is more common in young people. Symptoms are large amounts of urine from 5 to 10 liters, which are passed in twenty-four hours commonly by these young people. The urine is free of sugar and albumin. These youths feel thirsty, have weakness, very little energy, and dry skin. Origin in almost half of all cases is unknown. Trauma to the head, which causes damage to the pituitary or a tumor in that area, causes the remainder of cases.

Treatment: Eradication of the causative factor if determined. When not due to specific injury of the pituitary, the disease is easily controlled by use of vasopressin replacement therapy. This may be given by injection or nasal spray.

Juvenile onset is diabetes that has its onset prior to the age of fifteen years, where the essential abnormality is related to absolute deficiency. This form usually is quite difficult to regulate.

Diabetes latent is diabetes mellitus that manifests itself during times of stress, such as pregnancy, infectious disease, obesity, or trauma. Previous to the stress, no clinical or laboratory findings of diabetes are present. There is a very strong possibility that such individuals will eventually develop overt diabetes mellitus.

Diabetes mellitus is a disorder of carbohydrate metabolism, characterized by hyperglycemia and glycosuria and resulting from inadequate production or utilization of insulin. Basic cause is still unknown. But direct cause is failure of beta cells of the pancreas to secrete an adequate amount of insulin, the result of a genetic disorder. But it may also result from a deficiency of beta cells caused by inflammation, malignant invasion of the pancreas, or surgery. In the absence of insulin, glycogenesis and glycolysis are adversely affected. It is currently thought that insulin acts primarily at the cell membrane, facilitating transport of glucose into cells.

Symptoms: Principal symptoms are elevated blood sugar (hyperglycemia) sugar in urine (glycosuria), excessive urine production (polyuria), excessive thirst (polydipsia), and increase in food intake (polyphagia). Urine contains diacetic acid, beta-hydroxybutyric acid, acetone when disease process is in advanced stage. More common in women and after the age of forty. Increased thirst, frequent urination, itching frequently about the genitals. Fasting blood sugar above normal range of 90 to 120mg/100ml of blood, boils, and carbuncles, vascular changes may be present. Loss of weight, emaciation, weakness, and debility. When severe diabetes is allowed to progress without proper treatment, coma occurs with weakness and sweet odor of breath; nausea, headache, vomiting, dyspnea, sense of intoxication, delirium, and deep coma, resulting to death.

Complications: diabetic acidosis due to excessive production of ketone bodies, low resistance to infections, those involving extremities and ulceration of lower extremities, increase in incidence of toxemia in pregnancy, cardiovascular and renal disorders, disturbances in electrolyte balance, eye disorders, such as blindness.

Prognosis: Diabetic is a chronic, incurable disease, but symptoms can be ameliorated and life prolonged by modern treatment. The isolation and eventual production of insulin in 1921 by Canadian physicians Banting and Best made it possible to allow persons with the disease to lead normal lives.

Treatment

Consists of diet, insulin, exercise, and hygienic measures. At first, the person should be placed on a well-balanced diet adequate in all basic essentials: carbohydrates, proteins, fats, vitamins, minerals and fluids. In many people, this may be all that is required. It is important that obese people with diabetes be placed on a diet that will help them lose weight. Control of diabetes is much more difficult in an obese person. Blood sugar determinations should be made at frequent intervals. For the reader's information, blood sugar and glucose are considered to be the same. When a person is given an adequate diet and practices exercises or daily activities and glucose still appears in the urine, insulin may be necessary. Its use is not required in every case and may be dangerous if not properly given. Drugs have been given by mouth for control of mild cases of diabetes. These have been used with success mostly in middle-aged and older people who still have some beta cells function.

DIET

Diet: Standardization of affected people is a balanced diet of approximately 1,000 to 1,200 calories may be recommended. The diet is modified according to the weight of the person. According to my experience, experiments, and research, a good diet or permanent healthy eating of good, nutritious, organic, natural, fresh foods from the ground, land animals raised and living free in the land like two to three decades before and still existing if people searched for them will do the trick for diabetic sufferers, especially for people with type 2 diabetes and other diseases also. What I suggest is a diet or food intake of all food groups without exception.

EXAMPLE: Complex carbohydrates such as grains should be the most. It should be vegetables, fruits, fiber, starch, protein from plants: tofu, soy, nuts, seeds, almond, beans, legumes, and animal protein moderately. Fats and sweets should be used sparingly. Dairy should be used very little and fat free, reduced fat, or 1 percent to up to 2 percent only for their minerals such as calcium, potassium, phosphorous, iron, zinc, and water. From all the food group, the individual can find the daily allowance of vitamins: B12, B-complex, etc., C, A, D, K, and all the enzymes, the hormones, and all the body's good juices for fluids and electrolytes balance. And don't forget water seven to eight eight-ounce glasses or cups in twenty-four hours daily.

TYPE 2 DIABETES

There is no way that you will know for sure if you have diabetes type 2 without testing yourself. You can't rely on one yearly visit to the doctor or annual checkup to really know that you are diabetic. Because of what follows, you will see what I mean:

1. *People usually go to the doctor after they eat breakfast and or snack, lunch, and dinner, definitely a meal or two depending on their appointment time.*

2. *The blood culture has been sitting in a metal container for hours before pickup and the technician will travel several miles before bringing it to the laboratory. And in the laboratory, the blood is not being tested until later.*

3. *It is also possible to have an elevated blood sugar for many reasons besides diabetes such as drugs like steroid and other conditions like being under pressure, stress, adrenaline, or other hormonal problem.*

Example: Prep for Employment Number 1

Many times I had to collect lab work for new employees, and some of their lab results, especially blood glucose, came back abnormal, which can become a lost opportunity for a good job. Therefore, what I do is request the lab slip with all the requirements and walk to the lab myself, get the blood taking, wait for the result, make a copy for the individual to keep, and bring back the lab result to be placed in the new employee's record. That is, if I worked in a facility with a laboratory. If the workplace does not have a lab and the blood has to be sent out, then I usually request the lab sleep with all the requirements, give it to the person to be tested, and tell him or her to take it to the nearest lab to be tested ASAP and return to the employment place. Almost always, I was right because everything came back normal and the person got the job.

Self-Testing

To me, everybody diagnosed with type 2 diabetes after a few visits should buy two different brands of glucometer and test themselves: when they wake up, before meals, and at bedtime with one drop of blood in both machines at the same time to make sure and notice the difference. Almost never will you find the same number in both machines. Sometimes the numbers can be very close. One day, I had tested one drop of blood in four different machines and the same drop of blood with a result different from each other such as 88, 94, 98, 99 before meal. After a woman traveled four miles without eating, she waited a half hour in the clinic before being called. By the time she got to the consultation table, her blood glucose went up to 300 and her blood pressure went up high to 140/88. Since she was tested by the medical assistant, I requested that the doctor retest her in my presence for both results. As an excellent professional, he did even better than I asked. He changed the glucometer, blood pressure machine, with a larger-size gauge. I watched him take both tests and let me take them too. We both got the same results, which were blood glucose 96, blood pressure 120/80.

With some diseases like diabetes, hypertension, and high cholesterol, you have to know about them and know how to test yourself, how to read the results and their meanings, how they change according to time of the day, what you eat, how much sleep and rest you have, how much stress you are under, your mood, if you are upset, if you had an argument before or after the test, which can change the results drastically.

A diagnosis of any one of these diseases should take at least two to three months of follow-up before confirmation and permanent treatment. Some people can have a usual blood sugar before meal of 70 to 99 and after meal between two to three hours a result of 100 to 199 the most. But that same people on some occasions have an above 200, which they can bring down with one-half to one hour of brisk walk or any one of the aerobic exercises. The same goes for high blood pressure or hypertension. Bad diet, overweight, lack of sleep or rest, being upset, having a lot of stress, taking some drugs can all change your normal blood pressure result to an abnormal one. From 110/70 or 120/80 when under crisis can change to 160/90 or even more which you can bring down with meditation, yoga, imagery, deep breathing exercises, relaxation, listening to music, having a good laugh with loved ones, and not having to take a pill with side effects. If you have a good doctor, I am sure he or she can tell you what to do besides taking medication or together with medication if it turns out to be serious. Because most of the time they are temporary and inaccurate. Most of the time, these two diagnoses are derived from side effects of some drugs or state of mind and almost never from diseases.

What I realized almost thirty years ago is that medicine is not an exact and accurate science like physics, mathematics, chemistry, astronomy, and astrology while anatomy, physiology, bacteriology, epidemiology, and some others are changeable and are rarely different in nature. The normal most of the time is just a number of people or things that are the same way most of the time. Also because some scientists made some kinds of discovery and pronounced it as normal and good while the others are abnormal and bad. They don't realize that there are other extremes that are good too but different occasionally. Therefore, these people with different results than the "normal" according to these scientists' discovery can mess up their good health by trying to move to the normal and have the normal test results. By doing this, they can be miserable and even sicker than before. I have so many examples for the above mentioned, I will only give three.

Example Number 2

In 1989, a handsome young fellow, well built, six feet four with lean muscles, weight 180 pounds, light skinned and with light brown eyes from the Caribbean, came to my polyclinic for annual checkup or physical. One of the nurses sent him immediately to the emergency room in the hospital. He insisted that all his life he has been like that since early childhood. And every time he went to a new doctor's office, the same thing happens. The entire staff refused to listen to the man. I asked them, "Why don't you listen to him?" There are many exceptions in almost everything in life. That's my belief. This man collected his entire lab, worked and tested results for the past ten years and never took the advices and suggestions of the new doctors or nurses. To me, people have to listen, be open to versatility, individual differences, and other options and have in mind that there is never one way for almost anything. Paying attention, listening, understanding, trying to be open and knowing that there are endless possibilities and probabilities for almost anything to happen should be a wise person belief. Like this young man who was supposed to die in a few minutes unless he had a blood transfusion, demonstrated that he could do several push-ups and sit-ups in a few minutes and went to the treadmill without being tired or having difficulty breathing, proved everybody at the clinic were wrong. Nevertheless, everybody was screaming, "No, sir, no, you can't do that, you are going to die." I was the only person encouraging and complimenting him for his courage, his admirable fitness and bravery due to what he has to go through all his life. His condition was a very low blood pressure and low blood cell count or anemia.

Example Number 3

I HAVE A GIRLFRIEND

I have a girlfriend since early childhood, and her mother who died at the age of ninety-two was diagnosed with type 2 diabetes since she was a young adult and got married and gave birth to eight children later on who became adults and great-grandparents themselves. Approximately ten years ago, during the annual physical, my girlfriend was diagnosed with type 2 diabetes and prescribed oral medications. She told her mother who then told her, "Don't listen to the doctors. Do like me who is eighty-two years old and was diagnosed since eighteen years old and never took one single pill all my life and still in perfect health. Just cook your own good foods, follow me with a good diet, activities, sleep well at night, and decrease stress." Once you start taking medication, you can't stop them because they are like crack cocaine, and you are going to need more and more until you will need insulin injection many times a day like a junkie. Unfortunately, she did not listen to her mother and she regretted it. Before the mother died from old age, my girlfriend told her mom, "You are correct in your prediction and I should've listened to you." At present, my girlfriend is taking several injections of insulin per day, can't even cook, clean after herself, take care of her grooming, and take care of continuing education and update her skills to keep up with technology in order to hold on to her income tax, insurance manager, and travel agency corporation. She looks older than her dead ninety-two-year-old mother. It's a must that you know your body better than anyone else. You need to have some knowledge in the medical science. You also need to know that medicine is not an exact science like physics, chemistry, astrology, astronomy, and mathematics. In our body, there is a threshold for some of our senses, such as taste, touch, etc., while in medicine there is a parameter for almost everything.

Examples:

- *Pulse from 60 to 84 with all the numbers in between is good, and 72 is the best. All of these results are normal.*
- *Temperature or body temperature that is 97.8 to 99.8 is good. But 98.6 is the best and all in between are normal.*
- *Blood pressure systolic or the number on top (since you have two main numbers) is from 100 over 140 and all in between numbers*

are good and normal depending on the person's age. But 120 is perfect or best in adults to old age.

- *The diastolic (which is the bottom number; 60 to 88 are good) 80 is perfect. This parameter goes for age, sex, and time of the day.*

Now you can see why diabetes is the fastest-growing disease in America. You can be an extreme or just different from the so-called normal person. You can have a trauma in your life, you can have a bacterial infection, depression, get very upset, angry, enraged, taking steroids prescribed for cellulitis, asthma, skin infection, arthritis, or any type of hormonal therapy for skin disorders or even acetaminophen or other painkiller that create liver problems or just releasing cortisol, the bad stress hormone and with all the above can change your blood glucose to an abnormal elevation temporarily. And blood pressure systolic elevations that will go down with time, your body system's own time, gaining weight or obesity can make you a diabetic. But if you don't know these facts and wait for the body's natural process and run to the doctors, you can become a statistic for diabetes and hypertension, which we will talk about later on. If you are obese, losing twenty pounds or more by following a good nutritious healthy diet and exercise daily can make your diabetes and hypertension something of the past. Therefore, read, research, experiment, use good judgment, and save yourself. Because today, a drug can be the best for a disease and the next day recalled for the poison it is made of. And you can also watch on TV all the lawyers to consult after your loved ones die because they used these drugs.

If your blood sugar or glucose is consistently elevated in your bloodstream, meaning no matter what you eat, how long you eat, before you eat, after you eat, with daily exercise, walking, drinking seven to eight eight ounces of water in twenty-four hours, taking medication or not; then it's about time to take action and do what you can, seek help, and get treated. Untreated diabetes can cause kidney failure, heart disease, blindness, and poor circulation in the lower extremities, which often require amputation of toes, legs, feet, or the whole leg.

Type 2 diabetes can be prevented, ameliorated, or stopped with lifestyle change; good eating habits; eating good food, nutritious food with all the needed vitamins, minerals; decreasing stress; exercises; activities; and avoiding complications in your life and keeping busy physically, emotionally, and spiritually with a network of friends, family, education, and a good support system. Although there is a claim that diabetes and other blood diseases are unnoticeable or have no signs or symptoms, I say no to that. There are signs and symptoms that can make some people seek help besides blood glucose testing.

These signs are as follows:

Tingling in your extremities, for example, hands, fingers, feet, and toes.
Blurred vision like a veil on top of your eyes.
Gum bleeding, which can lead to infection even with good dental care.
Fatigue, not just feeling tired after hard work, but feeling tired all the time.
Lack of concentration.
Unable to solve usual problems that were not so difficult in the past.
Weight loss or gain against your will that you can't explain and can't stop even with diet and exercise.
And for women who are having vaginal yeast infection too often can be a sign of diabetes.

Later on, there are other signs such as the three Ps, which are the following:

Polyphasia: Eating too much or a lot
Polyuria: Urinating often or a lot more than one liter per night.
Polydipsia: Drinking a lot of water or too much or more than eight eight ounces of water in less than two-four hours.

The 3 Ps: hunger, thirst, urinating too much or too often.

The urine sometimes can have pieces of hard sugar, ketone, or acid for acidosis that turn the blue litmus paper red, make your mouth taste sour. If you happen to see a doctor, there are tests he or she can administer to find out if you have diabetes and send you for laboratory test.

To prevent, avoid, or eliminate this disease, do the following: have a diet that contain fruits, vegetables, dried beans of any color, legumes, whole grains, lean protein, and fat-free or low-fat dairy product. Have multiple small meals or snacks between each meal such as breakfast, lunch, and dinner of small to moderate size. Make sure that your best protein is from *animals, such as poultry, fish, or lean meat of serving the size of the palm of a child. Because you need the plant protein from nuts, almond, beans, tofu, soy, rice, and beans combination and whole grains. A serving of rice and pasta (cooked) should be one-half of an eight-ounce cup that is a four-ounce cup. You also need a four-ounce cup or bowl of fruit pieces you cut yourself right from the farm or supermarket or as fresh as you can. The same goes for fresh vegetables that you steamed and fresh salad daily from your own garden or farm and supermarket. Stay away from processed foods, canned foods, sugary or concentrated sweet foods, juices that contain high-fructose corn syrup, corn syrup, sodas, and candy. Use only the sweet in the food naturally.*

Please do not replace your fresh fruits and vegetables serving with juices even if the juices are 100 percent natural because the fruits and vegetable as a whole contain fiber that slow down the absorption of sugar that they contain into the bloodstream. While juices have less fiber and activate the process of sugar absorption in the bloodstream that causes the blood sugar levels to rise rapidly. Therefore, eat your fruits, vegetables, and salads as whole or pieces raw or steamed and enjoy their savory flavors, their high fiber content that can prevent the risk of having diabetes or reduce the progress if you already have it.

Precaution: if you already have diabetes, make it a habit to check your blood pressure also. Know what your blood pressure should be. Check your blood pressure parameter on the page that applies to blood pressure and buy a self-testing blood pressure machine with explanations on how to do it easily. Check your blood pressure twice a day, in the morning and afternoon while testing your blood sugar or glucose even if you test your blood sugar many times a day. Make sure that with the early morning and early evening you check your blood sugar and blood pressure and record the reading in a logbook. If you don't want to buy a blood pressure device, you can check your blood pressure at the drugstore near the pharmacy in a department store or grocery store where most of them have a pharmacy inside. It's easy to do by yourself or some pharmacy's employees would be glad to help you. Because according to some scientists, researchers, and my own research, these two diseases for some unfortunate reason unknown to me and some researchers often go together. It also seems to me that there is a third brother who is appearing in addition to the two previously mentioned, which is high cholesterol LDL level (the fatty cholesterol) and triglycerides. We will talk about that in another chapter. Just know that combination can cause heart attack or heart disease and stroke. When you have your annual checkup, have your doctor send you to a laboratory for a complete blood count with differential, chemistry, and lipid profile, in other words the whole things and ask for a copy of the tests result. Work on your own with testing, good habits, good foods, exercises to prevent these three conditions from settling in your body.

TREATMENT

People with diabetes usually suffer from nerve damage that disguise their feelings of irritation, cuts, bruises, and other foot problems. These people should have a daily inspection of their feet for swelling, redness, discolorations, and small cuts. They should wear good and well-fitted shoes indoor and outdoor. They should wear different shoes every day and never wear the same pair of shoes for two days in a row to prevent the risk of bacterial and fungal infections. They should wash their feet with warm water and mild liquid soap or bars patted dry with a clean soft cloth towel or paper towel, moisturize them with a good lotion like Eucerin or Cetaphil or any good lotion free from dyes and a lot of chemicals or fragrance. When you are applying the moisturizer, skip between the toes because it can promote infections such as athlete's foot. The lotion can also soften the tissue and prevent drying out or cracking skin and tissues.

FOOD GOOD FOR DIABETES

Diabetes is the fastest-growing disease in America at the present. Therefore, we all need knowledge of what to eat to prevent it or to ameliorate it. You may never get it if you eat certain foods daily. These foods can prevent the risk of diabetes up to 21 percent or lower, according to research, experiments, and statistics.

Make sure that you are not allergic to peanuts first then eat a spoonful of peanut butter a day to lower your risk of having diabetes. If you already have diabetes, it can lower the disease progression. Don't eat more than two tablespoons daily because of calories, sugar, salt, and fat. Make sure you read all labels before you buy peanut butter and all other prepared foods. Better yet, buy your roasted, unsalted, and unshelled peanuts and your own food processor machine. Then make your all-natural and organic peanut butter.

CASE STUDY 31

While in my last year in my master's degree in education, I had an African lady as teacher for four different classes. Therefore, we became acquainted. She used to eat a small bowl of peanut butter that she made herself lunch and a mango for dessert. She always looked healthy, strong, physically fit, and also in a good mood. Contrary to some people's beliefs, peanut butter does not make people fat. Peanut butter can cut triglycerides in your blood. Triglycerides are fat that can cause heart disease and stroke. And this teacher knew that much.

Therefore, don't hesitate to eat a peanut butter sandwich made with whole grain or whole-wheat bread for lunch or snack. Peanut butter is also good for many other diseases. Peanut or peanut butter can help you lose weight, reduce your bad LDL cholesterol, and prevent bone loss. We will talk about peanut butter and other diseases or conditions later in another chapter alphabetically. Eat food that lower your glycemic index because these foods can lower your risk of having diabetes or reverse it if you already have it. Try to have most of your daily calories from fruits and vegetables. Eat foods with lots of fibers because fibers slow down the release of sugar into your bloodstream. Foods such as brown rice or other colors, dried beans, lentils, oats, whole-grain breads and pastas can help too. Avoid foods made with white rice, flour, potatoes, and some cereals made with less fiber.

According to some studies, one to two cups of coffee a day any way you want, such as decaffeinated, with caffeine, black, with low-fat milk, low-fat cream, and sugar added can help reduce the risk of diabetes type 2. According to me or my experience, do not drink more than two cups a day due to the side effects of caffeine, xanthine, thiothixine, and other elements in coffee. Researchers are not sure why coffee can decrease insulin resistance.

To me, anyway, one cup or two of coffee a day can be good for many things, for example, constipation because of the warm or hot liquid, clearing your mind or foggy brain, keeping you awake and energetic to start the day. Therefore, if you don't have something to prevent you from drinking coffee, drink a cup or two a day.

The purpose of this chapter is not so much to cure, but to prevent people from having this dreadful condition. I would suggest that people ask their caregiver to test their blood sugar at yearly visits and at any age, especially if their weight increases to ten or more pounds in one year and if they have it in their family, they are not active in a gym or other exercises. There is a possibility that many people can be a prediabetic or full diabetic and don't even know it.

For many years, I had never heard of prediabetes. It was either you are a diabetic or not. But recently due to obesity, there is a condition called prediabetes that several millions of Americans suffer from.

Anyone with a fasting blood sugar between 100 and 125 in a few tests is a prediabetic. This condition can be stopped from progressing to diabetes type 2, if you know of it early and take action. We all know by now, 2013, how devastating this disease can be. And a large percent of prediabetes is bound to develop to full diabetes with the risk of having a cohort of other conditions such as kidney failure, blindness, heart diseases, circulatory problems, which can lead to amputation and stroke. I urge you if you are reading this part of the book to lose a few pounds according to how heavy you are, overweight, or obese to go get some activities, get a doctor or nurse to test your blood sugar level at different times of the day. Better yet, buy your own glucometer and test yourself daily and write down the result in your log book and take it to the doctor. Also, practice what is in this book about foods to eat and not to eat. This book alone can help you not to develop prediabetes or not develop at all if you are already a prediabetic, or it will take you at least twenty-six years or more to become a full diabetic by neglecting your good habits instead of just a few months.

For people who are prediabetic or full type 2 diabetic among all the other good foods in this book, broccoli is the number one food that can prevent, reverse, and heal all the damages done to your blood vessels. Therefore, eat broccoli cooked or raw as a snack or meal and benefit from the compound name sulforaphane, which stimulates production of enzymes that protect blood vessels and decrease the level of free radical molecules that destroy all kind of cells in your body including blood cells. This is a fact, according to scientists and researchers.

I really don't know what more to do to emphasize the risks of type 2 diabetes to people. Therefore, I don't mind repeating to myself. According to statistics, everyday news, surveys, researches in 2008, diabetes type 2 in the United

States alone had reached epidemic proportions with a wrapping number of 24.8 million people who have the full disease and 56.8 million people with the new condition called prediabetes, which left untreated can turn to full diabetes itself with a cohort of other diseases and conditions. I am not afraid to tell you that obesity is the number one culprit that triggers diabetes type 2. Therefore, people, you have to fight obesity and must lose weight. It is imperative that you do something about what you are eating, acquire knowledge on how to eat moderately some good foods, exercise, and be active. To me, people in general need to get up and "book" and not just walk but run like your tail is on fire. Please make a food and activity diary or log, be organized, have some good sleep, not so much rest and sitting down but being in bed sleeping for a decent number of hours from seven to eight hours per night. You probably ask why. The answer is when you are sleeping, your level of hunger raises and produce the bad hormone name ghrelin. And you don't want to do anything else but eat sweet, salty, and fatty foods. In turn, your risk for type 2 diabetes increases. Therefore, sleep enough because when you sleeping, you can't eat anyway. If you have problem sleeping, do the following:

1. Get your room at a temperature of seventy-two degrees Fahrenheit. And arrange to make it dark and cozy.
2. Don't do any extra-hard activities three to four hours before bedtime.
3. Clear your mind of problems and stop thinking of anything.
4. Wear your comfortable sleepwear.
5. Go to bed, take five deep breaths, relax, and go to sleep.
6. When you wake up, don't skip breakfast or the first meal and do not make food for lunch or dinner as your first meal. Because when you do, this exchanges the mealtimes especially for diabetics, who are more likely to become obese, according to scientists and my own experiment.
7. Have fiber foods and lean protein, enough vitamin D, calcium and vitamin C in your food list of good foods for diabetic such as blueberries because they contain vitamin C and B and are rich in fibers, which can increase blood circulation and improve memory.

Flaxseeds

Flaxseed slows down glucose or sugar absorption, the major cause of diabetes. Therefore, sprinkle ground flaxseed or oil on your salads or oatmeal, which is already full of soluble fibers that can regulate sugar in your blood and insulin level from your pancreas by restraining the digestion of starches. Oatmeal can also lower your fatty cholesterol (LDL) level, preventing you from another culprit-causing diabetes.

SWEET PEPPERS

Green, red, yellow, and orange, it doesn't matter the color because they are all full of vitamin C, beta-carotene, and antioxidants (especially for people who can't eat fish, which protects your body and prevent you from having diabetes type 2 or fight it if you already have it).

SPINACH

This food is very rich in many good vitamins and minerals, which can boost your immune system and protect some of your vital organs from the ravages of diabetes. But if you already have type 2 diabetes, you need to test your blood sugar level before you eat a bowl of spinach alone or without other food as a meal. Because a bowl of spinach without other foods as a meal can drop your blood sugar level so fast and so low that it can cause a dangerous crisis.

WALNUTS

Walnuts are very good to reduce insulin-resistance hormones that control glucose levels. Walnuts also have omega-3 fatty acid, which is good for heart circulation, which causes problems for diabetics.

YOGURTS

Yogurts that are fat free or low fat, organic, all natural, free from chemicals, pesticide, and insecticides can strengthen your immune system, making you fight many diseases, especially diabetes.

DRY BEANS OR ANY BEANS

Beans of all colors doesn't matter because they are rich in fiber, which slows down sugar into your blood stream and stop glucose levels from soaring but stay even or regular.

TOFU

For people who are vegan or don't need too much animal fat in their diet, tofu can do the trick by providing plant protein to them and increase their needed level of insulin.

PUMPKIN

Pumpkin contains a lot of antioxidants and another substance called D-chiro-Inositol, which can boost insulin production and help diabetes in both types, which are type 1 and 2, according to some research and experiments.

SALMON

Salmon provides a lot of omega 3 that can slow down artery diseases in people with type 2 diabetes.

The rest of the diseases will be continued in another book. Thank you.

ABOUT THE AUTHOR

There are three subjects in this world that I choose not to ever discuss in my life: beauty, politics, and religion.

Here is why:

Beauty: For almost every mother in the world, their sons and daughters are the most beautiful children or persons in the world. For almost every lover or romantic persons in the world, the person he or she is in love with is the most beautiful person in the world!!!!

Politics: For almost every politician in the world, no matter how defective or unqualified, the politician believes their party is the best. Although I am not affiliated with any political party, I still vote privately as a citizen.

Religion: For almost every religious person in the world, he or she believes that his or her religion is the true, the real, the most perfect worldwide religion or cult.

And who am I to say otherwise???

For me, what is important is not what comes through your mouth, but what stays in your head, mind, heart, and soul.

To me, searching and making sure of what you say or do in detail and early enough is always a useful quality. One of my biological children always tells me when she confides in me that I always take things to the extreme. She always tells me, "Just listen until I finish talking before you tell me what to do." Most of the time, by her first sentence, I tell her the answer or what to do.

For example, what I am writing about now, "cancer", in March 15, 2014, are my notes of what I have observed and known since March 1998, which means how early people should take cancer and almost all other diseases seriously.

Back to my daughter and thanks to text messages, instead of calling and listening, she texts the questions or stories, and I text back the answers in detail for her to understand without interruption. Then she replies, "Good" or "Great answer, thank you, Mom!" I said, "You are always welcome, my love!!"

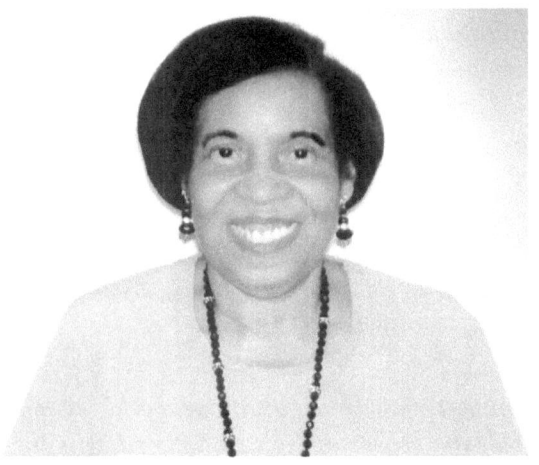

Earth Brother

Not too long ago, I did an experiment. I went to the nearest mall from my house. I found a large group of teens of different ages, races, and complexion, but they were all males. They were loud, unorganized, and risky. But regardless of the danger, instead of calling security like some other people might have done, I approached them. I picked one of them who was close to my size and hugged him and said, "You are my brother and I love you." His response was, "Lady, who are you? I am a little boy. I don't know you and don't live in this neighborhood." I said, "But you are a human being living in America, on a planet named Earth in the same century." He said, "Yes." I replied, "I am an old lady doing the same thing, isn't it great?" He exclaimed, "Yes!!!" The others said yes also. I continued my usual hour walk and met them back and forth, and each time we met, they said, "The earth century sister, we love you." I said, "I love you too. Be good, be healthy, and live to the next century."

I am very creative. I almost always have ideas, creations, and inventions, which I use often when I work in construction for myself and family. I do decorating, arts and crafts, painting, and sewing. I made my own tools, which were very becoming because they worked beautifully for my needs.

I like to research, observe, experience, and experiment all throughout my life. I love to be my own scientist. I listen, investigate, and read statistics in newspapers, books, magazines, and other media. I put two and two together and experiment with the information in order to create my own ideas, opinions, and theories.

Qualifications

- *Registered nurse.*
- *Certificate in Food Protection from the New York City Department of Health.*
- *Certificate from the New York State Department of Health Division of Nutrition Child and Adult Care Food Program (created by the Department of Agriculture).*
- *Certificate in Infection Control from the New York State Department of Health*
- *Certificate from the New York State Office of Alcoholism and Substance Abuse Services from the Academy of Addiction Studies.*
- *Certificate from the American Association of Professional Hypnotherapists.*
- *Degrees in psychology, nursing, and education.*
- *Diplomas from business school, sponsored by the government for business administration and legal and executive secretary and stenography.*
- *I also have many more diplomas and certificates for the thirty-eight years of higher education studies at various universities in the United States alone, without studies done abroad.*
- *In 2008, I had my first book* T.H.A.T.S., The Health Assistance to Some *published.*